THE SALT OF THE EARTH
    can help put you six feet under

SUGAR IS SWEET
    —but not as sweet as staying alive

LET'S HAVE ANOTHER CUP OF COFFEE
    —and raise your blood pressure another notch

SMOKE GETS IN YOUR EYES
—but what it does to your veins is murder

All these substances—and others whose effects Carlson Wade describes—have been shown to raise blood pressure and contribute to heart attacks, strokes, and circulatory conditions. Drawing on medical and nutritional expertise from many sources, Mr. Wade shows how to do without these substances, substituting natural products which enhance, not endanger, your health.

FACT/BOOK
ON
Hypertension (High Blood Pressure) and Your Diet

Carlson Wade

Keats Publishing, Inc. New Canaan, Connecticut

FACT/BOOK ON HYPERTENSION AND YOUR DIET
Pivot Original Health Edition published 1975
Copyright © 1975 by Carlson Wade

Printed in the United States of America

Library of Congress Catalog Card Number: 74-31668

PIVOT ORIGINAL HEALTH BOOKS are published by
Keats Publishing, Inc.
36 Grove Street
New Canaan, Connecticut 06840

ACKNOWLEDGMENT

Gratitude is extended to the High Blood Pressure Information Center of the National Institute of Health for the use of their charts, graphs and lists as they appear in this book. Material obtained from sources other than the U.S. Department of Health, Education and Welfare are so acknowledged.

CONTENTS

The Effects of High Blood Pressure

Persistent high blood pressure damages the cardiovascular system—the heart and blood vessels. This system may be compared to a tree. The largest artery—the aorta—is the trunk. The aorta carries blood from the heart to be distributed by branch arteries to all parts of the body. The smallest arteries, called arterioles, are the twigs. The walls of the arterioles are normally elastic, but under sustained high blood pressure they harden and lose their flexibility. This may happen naturally with age, but high blood pressure hastens the process. To overcome this resistance, the heart pumps harder and in time is unable to keep up with the demands made upon it. The hardening of the arteries also increases the likelihood that a blood clot will interfere with the normal flow of blood to the heart, brain, kidney, or other organ. The result may be one of the disabling and often fatal complications of high blood pressure—a heart attack, a stroke, or kidney failure.

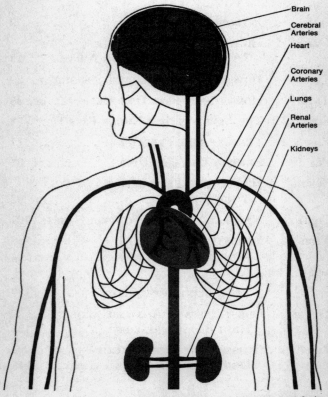

Brain

Cerebral Arteries

Heart

Coronary Arteries

Lungs

Renal Arteries

Kidneys

Source: National Institute of Health U.S. Public Health Service

INTRODUCTION

High blood pressure, or hypertension, is one of the nation's major health problems because it can lead to fatal heart diseases and cerebral strokes. It is a serious health problem because it is sneaky, often undetected, with few, if any, apparent symptoms. It can increase in severity, unnoticed, until it causes a grave illness. This book will explain what hypertension is and how modern nutritional science is able to help control it, adding years of health to the lives of hypertensive people.

If you are told that you have hypertension, you may become suddenly frightened or bewildered. It is true that your Aunt Hattie or Uncle Mark might have died of a stroke, but when you relate hypertension to stroke, you are usually uncertain as to what kind of future you face.

This book will help shed light on the problem. Within the last few years, hypertension has been acknowledged as one of the leading health risks of our time. There is increasing emphasis upon the necessity to have your blood pressure checked since this symptomless ailment might not otherwise be detected.

To become acquainted with hypertension, let us look at the latest facts. The National Heart and Lung Institute estimates that 23 million Americans have high blood pressure. Hypertension kills 60,000 Americans a year. It creates such conditions as stroke and kidney failure which cause 1.5 million illnesses or deaths.

Generally, hypertension afflicts more women than men up to the age of fifty-five. The rate of occurrence is highest in blacks. According to 1971 estimates, hypertension was prevalent in 12.7 percent of white men and 17.3 percent of white women. Among blacks, 25.7 percent of the men and 28 percent of the women suffered from hypertension. Blood pressure tends to go up with age, and it levels off at about fifty-five. But it may go higher when you are subjected to tensions and errors in healthful living. This sneaky killer can creep up without warning.

Drug treatment has its limits since it causes side effects. Furthermore, experts say that only one out of every eight Americans with dangerously high blood pressure is taking drugs that offer any help. Half of the people with high blood pressure don't know they have it. Half of those who do know don't bother going to a doctor. And half of those who see a doctor eventually discontinue medication.

The reason for such a careless attitude is that high blood pressure causes very little discomfort. You may have dangerously high pressure, but your eyes won't pop, your blood vessels won't bulge. You'll feel great . . . until it's too late. This emphasizes the importance of learning about hypertension and how to use the newest programs for natural control.

The need for natural healers is most important since the average person is indifferent to a symptom-free ailment. There are other difficulties in drug therapy. If you take prescribed drugs for hypertension, you may have to pay over $500 a year to a physician; what you pay the pharmacy cannot even be calculated. Costs keep increasing. This is a lot of money for someone who is not conscious of his high blood pressure. He might even feel better after discontinuing treatment with its uncomfortable side effects. There is also the inconvenience of making regular doctor and/or clinic visits. But the very nature of high blood pressure calls for long-term treatment. Most physicians and hospital clinics are geared toward quick treatment—instant medicine—and cannot accommodate prolonged therapy for this ailment. Many doctors agree that the medical profession is not yet equipped to meet the public need for long-term hypertension treatment. The use of natural methods helps eliminate the cause, ease the reactions and make life longer and healthier.

The purpose of this book is to alert you to the hidden risks of hypertension and to the ways in which proper body care can help reduce or eliminate the incidence of strokes or cardiovascular ailments that might incapacitate or end your life.

Nature meant you to have a healthy body; good health has its roots in good blood pressure. Cooperate with Nature and your pressure can respond in kind.

CARLSON WADE

CHAPTER ONE

HIGH BLOOD PRESSURE . . . "A TIME BOMB TICKING AWAY . . ."

ABOUT ONE IN TEN OF ALL ADULTS IN THE world has high blood pressure, or hypertension, as it is known medically. The World Health Organization (WHO) calls high blood pressure "a widespread epidemic."

In the United States alone, it is a major contributing factor in an estimated 250,000 deaths and many of the more than 1,500,000 heart attacks and strokes that occur each year. Yet, once detected, this ailment can usually be effectively controlled.

Doctors estimate that some 23 million persons in the United States have high blood pressure. Half of them don't know they have it. Many of those that do know are not being treated effectively. High blood pressure is so symptomless that it has been compared to a "time bomb ticking away" in your body. When it goes off . . . it is too late for healing!

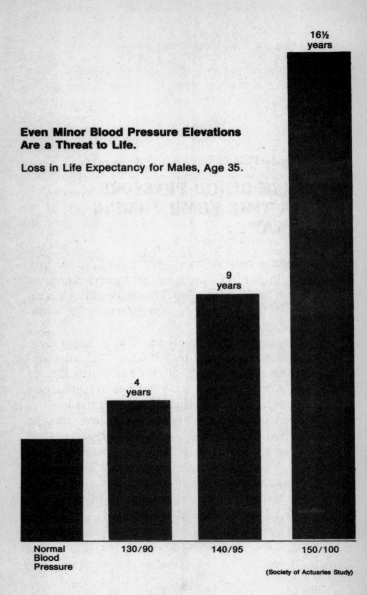

Even Minor Blood Pressure Elevations Are a Threat to Life.

Loss in Life Expectancy for Males, Age 35.

16½ years

9 years

4 years

Normal Blood Pressure | 130/90 | 140/95 | 150/100

(Society of Actuaries Study)

WHAT DOES "BLOOD PRESSURE" MEAN?

Blood pressure refers to the amount of pressure exerted in the bloodstream as it passes through the arteries. When the left ventricle of the heart contracts, or squeezes down, it forces the blood out into the arteries. The major arteries then expand to receive the oncoming blood. The muscular linings of the arteries resist the pressure; the blood is squeezed out into the smaller vessels of the body. The blood pressure is the combined amount of pressure the blood is under as a result of the pumping of the heart, the resistance of the arterial walls and the closing of the heart valves.

The maximum pressure in the arteries is related to the contraction of the left ventricle and is called the *systolic* pressure. The minimum pressure, which exists when the heart is at maximum relaxation, is referred to as the *diastolic* pressure.

Everyone needs blood pressure to move blood through the circulatory system. The pressure goes up and down within a limited range, but *when it goes up and stays up,* it is called high blood pressure. A systolic pressure of 150 and a diastolic reading of 95 (or 150/95) is generally considered high blood pressure. A normal reading would be about 120/80, although it is recognized that the definition of normal varies from person to person.

In some people, high blood pressure is associated with another ailment such as diabetes, a kidney disorder or tumors. But usually, no cause can be detected. Still, the risks are all too clear.

Hypertension places the heart and arteries under abnormal strain. Excess pressure constantly pounds the body organs fed by the blood supply. As a result,

High Blood Pressure More Than Triples the Risks of Heart Failure and Stroke.

Source: The Framingham, Massachusetts Heart Study

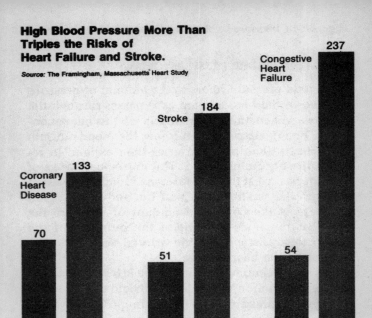

Coronary Heart Disease

Stroke

Congestive Heart Failure

70   133   51   184   54   237

| Normal | High | Normal | High | Normal | High |

Number of Patients with Normal and High Blood Pressure

Treatment Can Ward off Complications and Lengthen Life. (VA Study)

Occurrence of heart failure, stroke, and kidney complications in patients with mild to moderate high blood pressure

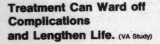

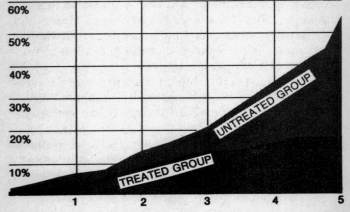

UNTREATED GROUP

TREATED GROUP

60%
50%
40%
30%
20%
10%

1   2   3   4   5

a blood vessel in the brain can burst, causing a stroke. Or the capacity of the kidney to filter wastes may be impaired. The heart, which must work harder to pump blood against the increased pressure in the arteries, may begin to show signs of strain. If ignored, high blood pressure can cause irreversible body damage.

WHAT IS HYPERTENSION?

Essential hypertension is a persistently elevated blood pressure—specifically, a diastolic pressure exceeding 95 millimeters of mercury—that cannot be attributed to any specific organic cause. Approximately 85 percent of all hypertension fits this definition. The other 15 percent is accounted for by various forms of *secondary hypertension,* which may result from:

Arteriosclerosis, or "hardening of the arteries." This ailment reduces the elasticity of affected arteries. Characteristic fatty deposits obstruct the bloodflow through them. Both of these factors tend to increase arterial blood pressure. Arteriosclerosis is often responsible for elevated blood pressure in elderly people.

Kidney diseases or obstructions to normal kidney bloodflow. These may cause the kidney to release renin into the blood. This enzyme catalyzes the formation of angiotensin from a plasma protein. A powerful blood-vessel constrictor, angiotensin is the most potent agent known for raising blood pressure.

Aldosteronism. This is a hormone that promotes the retention of salt and water by the kidneys and thus tends to expand plasma volume. Excessive secretion of this hormone may cause an increase in blood pressure.

Pheochromocytoma. This is a tumor associated with the adrenal glands. It is usually benign and seldom spreads to other parts of the body. But it produces and releases into the blood large quantities of the hormones norepinephrine and epinephrine. They raise blood pressure by stimulating the heart and constricting blood vessels.

Unlike essential hypertension, which can be controlled but not cured, secondary hypertension can often be cured if the underlying cause can be eliminated.

WHAT HAPPENS WHEN PRESSURE INCREASES?

Think of your heart, arteries and arterioles as a system of garden hoses that end in little nozzles (the arterioles). If you decrease the volume of spray from the nozzle, the hose becomes firm under increased pressure. It is under tension. Less water is flowing through, but it shoots out to a greater distance. Closing down the nozzle regulates the rate and pressure at which the water flows.

Something similar happens in hypertension. The arterioles tighten down; the heart has to work harder to pump blood through the tissues at a nearly normal rate. This maintains the pressure in the arteries and arterioles.

Arterial hypertension, or high blood pressure, is a dangerous ailment because of its effect on the walls of the arteries. It accelerates the ailment of atherosclerosis. Many people without high blood pressure have atherosclerosis; but those with high blood pressure have much more severe cases of the illness.

As we have said, the inside of a normal artery is quite smooth and flexible. There is plenty of room for the blood to flow through. However, in the later years of life, there is a tendency for the blood vessels to harden and the muscles to become less flexible.

THE EFFECTS OF ARTERIOSCLEROSIS AND CHOLESTEROL

When arteriosclerosis occurs in the vessels of the brain, the roughened spots on the vessel linings may cause the blood flowing over them to clot. Or the vessels may become partially or completely occluded; fatty deposits may weaken the vessel walls and rupture and bleeding result. In either case, part of the brain is injured and the person has an "apoplectic stroke."

Cholesterol is a complex, waxlike substance. An excess, along with other fatty substances, can become deposited in the walls of the blood vessels. This leads to atherosclerosis. The cells of the blood vessels react to cholesterol as to a foreign substance. Scar tissue is laid down around it to wall it off. It is this walling off that distorts and obstructs the normally smooth, round contour of the blood vessels and produces arteriosclerosis.

When excessive cholesterol obstructs the arteries, there is a great risk of high blood pressure. Furthermore, people with high blood pressure often not only have atherosclerosis but an ailment of the middle part of the artery wall called the "media." It is known that the atheroma (fatty substances), the scar formations of the lining of the arteries, as well

The Heart and Circulatory System

The heart is a four-chambered double pump that beats 100,000 times a day while moving 4,300 gallons of oxygen-rich blood through the circulatory system to the entire body.

As the heart beats, contractions of the thick muscle wall (myocardium) pump blood from the heart through 60,000 miles of blood vessels. The heart rests only a fraction of a second between beats. The normal adult circulatory system contains about eight pints of blood, which is recirculated continuously throughout the body.

The heart has two pumping stations. The right heart pump receives the blood after it has delivered nutrients and oxygen to the body tissues, then starts it on its journey to the lungs. The lungs cleanse the blood of waste gas (carbon dioxide) and provide it with a fresh supply of oxygen. The left heart receives this "recycled" blood from the lungs and pumps it through the circulatory system to its eventual return to the right heart.

This recycling process is activated by a small node in the upper right chamber of the heart—actually an electronic impulse center—that normally regulates the heart to 60 to 80 beats a minute. The node sends out electrical impulses which travel through the heart's own intricate nervous system. This is the power source, the heart's own "pacemaker."

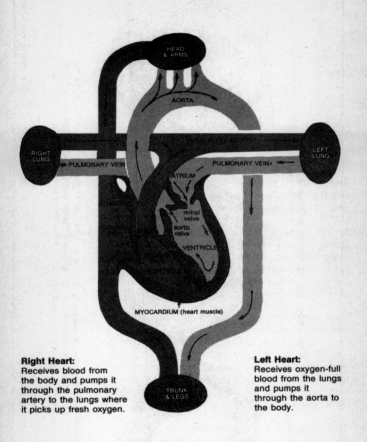

Right Heart:
Receives blood from the body and pumps it through the pulmonary artery to the lungs where it picks up fresh oxygen.

Left Heart:
Receives oxygen-full blood from the lungs and pumps it through the aorta to the body.

Your Heart and How it Works

Source: American Heart Association

The Progress of Atherosclerosis

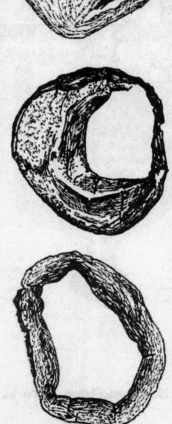

The deterioration of a normal artery (left) is seen as atherosclerosis develops and begins depositing fatty substances and roughening the channel lining (center) until a clot forms (right) and plugs the artery to deprive the heart muscle of vital blood which results in heart attack.

as the degeneration of the middle part of the artery wall concur with high blood pressure. There is a direct relationship between these factors and the duration and height of the blood pressure.

THERE IS NO WARNING

The absence of symptoms is one of the major problems in identifying high blood pressure and getting treatment under way. The condition offers no warnings. It works its damage slowly and quietly while you feel fine.

Many hypertensive people don't realize anything is wrong with them, and all too often, the first indication of trouble is a stroke or heart attack that might have been prevented had the condition been diagnosed and treated. United States statistics show the highest death rate from these ailments, with about 28 deaths per 100,000 population. The figure is growing.

Symptoms of trouble are not reliable clues. Headaches may be caused by hypertension, or they may simply indicate the need for new glasses. There may be dizziness, fatigue, heart palpitations or flushing of the face. But the only certain, typical change is in the blood pressure itself.

Headaches are the most common incapacitating symptom. They often are present on waking from sleep, but they may occur at any time of day. They do not signify that a hemorrhage in the brain is in the making; nor do they indicate that the blood pressure is exceptionally high. It may be exceptionally low! But consistent headaches are considered clues to increased blood pressure.

Dizziness, or lightheadedness, accompanies a

Arteries in Blood Pressure

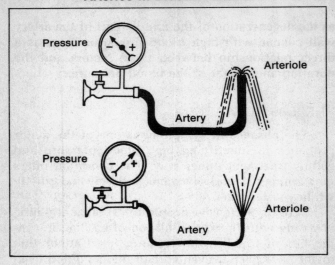

Factors Contributing to Essential Hypertension

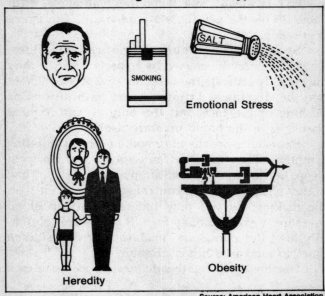

Source: American Heart Association

feeling of fullness in the head and tightness over the scalp, and may signal hypertension. Numbness and tingling in the arms and fingers are also associated with elevated blood pressure. Vertigo, a sensation that the world is moving about you, or that you are moving in space, is a more definite symptom. These are warning conditions.

SIX WAYS TO HELP HYPERTENSION

If your doctor has diagnosed hypertension, then cooperate with him in controlling this ailment. The American Heart Association, in *Your Blood Pressure* offers six helpful suggestions:

1. *Try not to worry.* Worry, nervous tension and emotional storms all help push up blood pressure.
2. *Keep your weight normal.* Overweight is a health hazard.
3. *Follow your doctor's advice on the use of tobacco and alcohol.* Smoking raises blood pressure in some people. Alcohol does not raise blood pressure; a moderate amount may even reduce it by releasing nervous tension. But some people react poorly to alcohol. Always follow your doctor's specific advice for you.
4. *Get plenty of sleep.* Take a short nap or two during the day if you can arrange it. Blood pressure is lowest during sleep and rises during waking hours.
5. *Choose sports that are not competitive.* Exercise is good for you, but avoid over-exertion at any time.
6. *Rest before you are tired.* You'll find that you

Risk Factors in Heart Attack and Stroke

These charts show the extent to which particular risk factors increased the risk of heart attack and stroke in the male population, aged 30–62 of Framingham, Massachusetts. For each disease, columns below the black horizontal line indicate lower than average risk; columns above the line, higher than average risk.

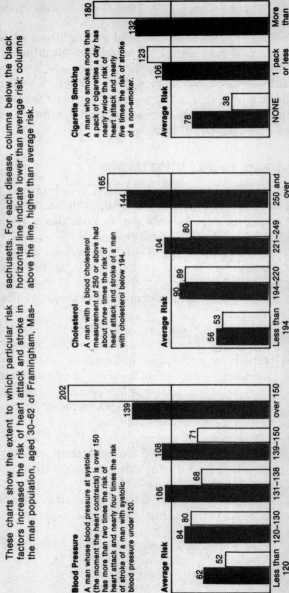

Blood Pressure

A man whose blood pressure at systole (the moment the heart contracts) is over 150 has more than *two* times the risk of heart attack and nearly *four* times the risk of stroke of a man with systolic blood pressure under 120.

Blood Pressure values:
- Less than 120: 62, 52
- 120–130: 84, 80
- 131–138: 105, 68
- 139–150: 108, 71
- over 150: 139, 202

Cholesterol

A man with a blood cholesterol measurement of 250 or above had about *three* times the risk of heart attack and stroke of a man with cholesterol below 194.

Cholesterol values:
- Less than 194: 56, 53
- 194–220: 90, 89
- 221–249: 104, 80
- 250 and over: 144, 165

Cigarette Smoking

A man who smokes more than a pack of cigarettes a day has nearly *twice* the risk of heart attack and nearly *five* times the risk of stroke of a non-smoker.

Cigarette Smoking values:
- NONE: 78, 38
- 1 pack or less: 106, 123
- More than 1 pack: 132, 180

The Danger of Heart Attack & Stroke Increases with the Number of Risk Factors Present

(example: 45 year old male)

This chart shows how a combination of three major risk factors can increase the likelihood of heart attack and stroke. For purposes of illustration, this chart uses an abnormal blood pressure level of 180 systolic, and a cholesterol level of 310 in a 45-year old man.

■ Heart Attack

□ Stroke (Atherothrombotic Brain Infarction)

Source: The Framingham, Massachusetts Heart Study

700

384

236

200

120

Average Risk

100

77 66

| NONE | cigarettes | cigarettes and cholesterol | cigarettes and cholesterol and blood pressure |

can do more in the long run. And you will avoid the tenseness and irritability that go with fatigue.

POINTS TO REMEMBER

When you analyze all of the studies and reports on high blood pressure and boil them down to a few short statements, this is what they say:

High blood pressure is very common—15 percent to 20 percent of the adult American population, or about 23 million people (the figure is growing) have the ailment.

High blood pressure is dangerous. It is a leading cause of stroke, heart disease, brain injury and kidney disease.

High blood pressure usually doesn't cause symptoms. The only way to know whether your blood pressure is high is to go to your doctor and have it read. The fact that you feel fine is no assurance your blood pressure is okay.

High blood pressure will cause the death of about 250,000 Americans in one typical year. That's five times the number of people who will be killed in auto accidents—or one out of eight of all people who will die from anything.

The National Health Examination Survey concluded that *hypertension is the most common chronic ailment in the United States.*

With these points in mind, let us see how blood pressure is measured, and how a natural approach to control can help you resist and correct irregularities.

CHAPTER TWO

HOW BLOOD PRESSURE IS MEASURED

BLOOD PRESSURE IS THE FORCE EXERTED against the walls of blood vessels by the blood flowing through them. This pressure is highest in the arteries and their finer branches called arterioles, drops sharply in the capillary bed, and is lower still in the veins returning "used" blood to the heart.

Blood pressure in the arteries supplying the body, or the systemic circulation, is considerably higher than that in the pulmonary arteries to the lungs. Unless otherwise specified, "blood pressure" refers to pressure in the arteries supplying the body.

Blood pressure is measured by an instrument called a *sphygomanometer* (Greek for pulse measurement). This is the procedure:

An inflatable armband with bulb attached is wrapped around your arm just above the elbow. When the bulb is squeezed, the armband fills with air, cutting off the blood flow in a large artery in the arm. At this point, the pressure from the armband on the artery is greater than the push of blood in the artery.

This pressure registers either on a dial attached to the armband or in an attached glass tube filled with mercury which has numbers marked on it, rather like a thermometer.

A stethoscope (the device used to hear heartbeats) is placed just below the armband on your arm.

As air is slowly let out of the armband, the level of mercury goes down. When the pressure in the band is less than the push of the blood in the artery, the beat of the blood as it is pushed by the heart through the artery is heard. The number on the dial or in the glass tube when the first beat is heard is noted. This shows the amount of pressure your heart exerts to pump blood, or how hard your heart is working; it is the *systolic* (upper) pressure.

As more air is let out of the band, it loosens. The blood starts to flow more steadily through the artery, and the beat is no longer heard. The number on the dial or in the glass tube at the point when the beat is no longer heard is also noted. This shows the least amount of pressure in your artery or how well your heart is relaxing; this is the *diastolic* (lower) pressure.

YOUR BLOOD PRESSURE IS
WRITTEN LIKE THIS:

Systolic pressure: Highest pressure produced by the heart when it is pumping blood.

Diastolic pressure: Lowest pressure in your blood vessels when the heart is relaxed.

Normal adult blood pressure should read:
Systolic under 140/diastolic under 90.

General guidelines: When recorded in a relaxed, resting person, normal systolic pressure is around

120, normal diastolic pressure is around 80. This would be written as 120/80. However, blood pressures somewhat above or below these values are also considered normal.

For example, a blood pressure of 140/90 is within the normal range, whereas 150/95 is a little high.

Systolic pressure tends to increase with age in healthy persons.

BASIC CAUSES OF HIGH BLOOD PRESSURE

If your doctor has diagnosed your pressure as being high, it may be traced to one or more of these basic causes, as outlined in *Your Blood Pressure* by the American Medical Association:

Diseases of the kidneys. In cases where the ailing kidneys can be healed, blood pressure almost always returns to normal.

Conditions affecting the adrenal glands. These two small but vital glands are located one on top of each kidney. Correction of the condition usually restores blood pressure to normal.

Localized narrowing of the aorta. This is a congenital defect in which a segment of the aorta (the body's largest artery) is narrowed. The heart must work harder to pump blood past the narrow point. The condition can be corrected and the blood pressure often returns to normal.

Defects in other arteries. Typical arteries that may have such defects are those that supply blood to the kidneys (renal arteries). These defects, too, are often correctable.

Disorders of the nervous system. These include infections of the brain (encephalitis) and brain

31

Blood Pressure Measurement

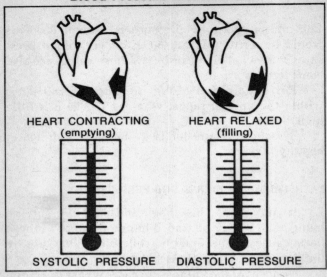

HEART CONTRACTING
(emptying)

HEART RELAXED
(filling)

SYSTOLIC PRESSURE

DIASTOLIC PRESSURE

Known Causes of Hypertension

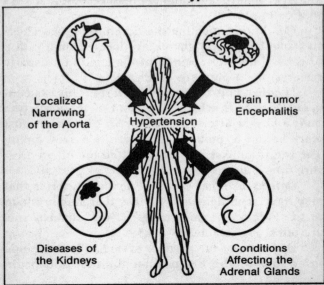

Localized
Narrowing
of the Aorta

Hypertension

Brain Tumor
Encephalitis

Diseases of
the Kidneys

Conditions
Affecting the
Adrenal Glands

Source: American Medical Association

tumors. Here, too, treatment is directed to the underlying cause.

Heredity factors. The AMA also explains that "essential hypertension occurs more commonly in people with a family history of high blood pressure. If one of your parents has the disease, there is a 50 percent chance that you or one of your brothers or sisters will develop it (usually between forty and sixty years of age). If both parents suffer from essential hypertension, the chance that one child will develop it rises to 90 percent.

"Although the cause of essential hypertension is not known, certain environmental factors are known to aggravate the condition in people who already have it. Among these are emotional tension (especially feelings of anger and frustration), large amounts of salt in the diet, cigarette smoking, and overweight."

VARIATIONS IN BLOOD PRESSURE READINGS

Every one's blood pressure goes up and down, not only with each heartbeat but also depending on whether they are awake or asleep, working hard or relaxing, excited or calm. So even a person whose range of blood pressure is normal most of the time can have temporary high blood pressure during stress.

But, in some people, for unknown reasons, blood pressure rises to unhealthy levels and doesn't come down even during rest. For this reason, the physician is interested in the level of your blood pressure during rest. He records it in his office while you are sitting or lying quietly.

Your blood pressure may go up after drinking

coffee, after an argument, after hearing some distressing news. It may go down within an hour. This fluctuation makes it essential to obtain regular readings. Again, it is to be emphasized that certain corrective living programs help to diminish a continuously high blood pressure.

HOW TO BEGIN CORRECTION OF HYPERTENSION

Any program has to begin with a complete physical and functional evaluation by a physician to determine whether a disease or malfunction of one of the organs of the body is responsible for the elevated blood pressure and if it can be corrected. He can make certain of the condition of the kidneys for instance, and test for several types of tumors.

Since sleep is the hypertensive's best friend, a brief period of bed rest may be a good beginning. Then, plan on nine hours of sleep a night, and learn to sleep or doze when the opportunity presents itself during the day—this can be a life-saving habit. If you cannot sleep, there is no harm in propping yourself up with a good book and reading. But be sure the book is not one that will excite you.

Except under special circumstances, moderate physical exercise should be part of the daily routine. Hard physical labor or any kind of physical exertion should be avoided, but mild exercise does not elevate blood pressure. Even during periods of heart failure, massage and light movement are necessary to help prevent blood clots from forming in the veins. But fatigue is a warning signal; so when exercising or playing a non-competitive sport, have the good sense to stop before you are tired.

Follow your physician's advice about your diet.

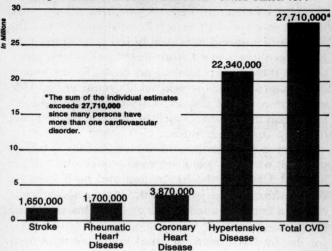

Estimated Prevalence of the Major Cardiovascular Diseases   United States: 1971

In Millions

*The sum of the individual estimates exceeds 27,710,000 since many persons have more than one cardiovascular disorder.

- Stroke: 1,650,000
- Rheumatic Heart Disease: 1,700,000
- Coronary Heart Disease: 3,870,000
- Hypertensive Disease: 22,340,000
- Total CVD: 27,710,000*

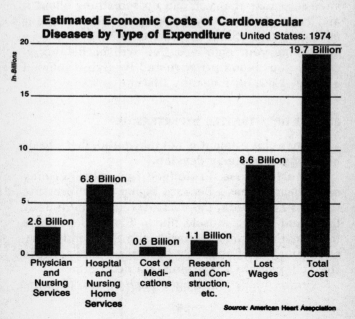

Estimated Economic Costs of Cardiovascular Diseases by Type of Expenditure   United States: 1974

In Billions

- Physician and Nursing Services: 2.6 Billion
- Hospital and Nursing Home Services: 6.8 Billion
- Cost of Medications: 0.6 Billion
- Research and Construction, etc.: 1.1 Billion
- Lost Wages: 8.6 Billion
- Total Cost: 19.7 Billion

Source: American Heart Association

Four light meals are better than three. Five or six lighter ones are even better. Food should be healthfully nutritious and not taken in too great quantities. If you are overweight, you must lose weight, since obesity must be avoided at all costs. Every pound of flesh means extra weight which requires just that many more blood vessels. This means more blood to nourish the tissues, which in turn forces the heart to pump that much harder.

Avoid stimulants—coffee, tea, alcohol, tobacco—that whip up your nervous system to further activity. Use caffeine-free coffee and herb teas. As for smoking, there is no doubt that a non-smoker stands a better chance for recovery in his battle for survival.

If you have been told that you have hypertension, recognize that you can do something about it and begin immediately by keeping calm. Nothing is more healing than a quiet, contented mind. By controlling your emotions, you will be helping to control your blood pressure and be giving yourself a longer lease on a healthy lifetime.

RESULTS OF UNTREATED HYPERTENSION

When this ailment is not diagnosed, these basic health problems may develop:

Heart disease. Prolonged hypertension may cause heart disease. Because higher blood pressure requires hard work, the heart develops abnormally thick and strong muscle fibers. Elevated pressure thickens the coronary arteries and they tend to become blocked. If an artery becomes completely obstructed, you are vulnerable to a heart attack.

Brain injury. Prolonged high blood pressure

frequently causes damage to the brain. A weakened vessel may rupture, causing an extensive hemorrhage. This may result in complete paralysis of one side of the body. A more common type of injury is a clot forming in an artery leading to the brain; this, too, can result in paralysis.

Visual disorders. Prolonged hypertension can produce serious changes in the eyes. A hemorrhage may occur which can interfere with the vision.

Kidney trouble. About one out of every two hypertensive patients eventually develop some trouble with their kidneys. This means frequent trips to the bathroom at night; albumin (a protein substance that is needed by the body but should *not* appear in the urine) may appear in the urine, indicating trouble with the filtering function of the kidneys.

In untreated hypertension, the time from onset to fatality is about twenty years. Except for an elevated blood pressure reading, no warning signs or symptoms are likely to appear for the first two thirds of this time, after which failure of one or more vital organs occurs. Once organ failure begins, the average survival of the untreated person is about six years.

Remember, it is your heart, your brain, your kidneys, and they're the only ones you've got. Don't underestimate their importance. Give yourself the consideration you deserve and your body the respect it deserves. Put your health first!

CHAPTER THREE

HOW A SALT-FREE DIET HELPS

A SALT-FREE DIET IS AN UNEXPECTEDLY PLEASant way to control high blood pressure. Without the use of the salt shaker, food tastes fresh and delicate, undisguised by the seasoning that often reduces varied flavors to a uniform sharpness. Abstaining from the use of salt in cooking, in seasoning and in processed commercial foods is of major importance in lowering blood pressure.

Frederick M. Allen, M.D. is credited with introducing a low salt diet for high blood pressure as far back as 1922. In the *Journal of the American Medical Association,* Dr. Allen explains that as a result of his twenty-eight years of experience with thousands of cases, the salt-free diet, especially when begun reasonably early, can definitely check hypertension.

"Whereas over 50 percent of persons with essential hypertension ordinarily die in congestive heart failure, and retinitis, claudication, angina and uremia are frequent, I have never witnessed a single onset of any of these complications in a patient on a continuous saltless diet."

A survey proved that eating salt contributes to hypertension. At a meeting of the American Society for Experimental Pathology, Dr. Lewis K. Dahl of the Brookhaven National Laboratory told of his findings in the cases of 448 patients. Of these, 55 were salt abstainers, 186 ate an average amount of salt and 207 sprinkled salt liberally on their food. Dr. Dahl emphasizes that there was no one with high blood pressure among the salt abstainers. There were 12 hypertensives in the intermediate group and 20 among those who used salt liberally. Dr. Dahl says this is not coincidence. He agrees with other medical specialists that salt is partly to blame for the development of high blood pressure. Or, to put it simply, the more salt you consume, the higher your blood pressure zooms.

Salt consumption often narrows the passageways of the small arteries. Salt may also whip up the action of the glands to secrete certain hormones that will also constrict the arteries, thus raising blood pressure. This is the finding revealed by Louis H. Nachum, M.D., in *Connecticut Medicine*. He found that by feeding high amounts of salt in the drinking water of test animals, there was a considerable increase in the blood pressure.

"If salt is involved in hypertension," says Dr. Nachum, "then the blood plasma of people with hypertension should contain more salt than the blood plasma of people with normal blood pressure. This was in fact found to be the case in a study made on a group of human patients."

The formula for salt is sodium chloride. Sodium is the villain as far as blood pressure is concerned.

Dr. Nachum says that if the sodium intake is gradually lowered to 400, 200 and 100 micrograms per day, then the average reduction in blood pressure can be 30 mm. systolic, and 16 mm. diastolic. "Less sodium can also reduce the size of the heart, cause the heart action to be more smooth and prolong life." Therefore, you can protect yourself against heart trouble and hypertension by eliminating the use of salt altogether, both in cooking and at the table.

Dr. Nachum cites cases of certain populations who consume little or no salt and know nothing of hypertension.

Basically, one of the main actions of this chemical (and it is a chemical!) is to cause swelling in the walls of the arterioles, those tiny arteries that carry fresh, oxygenated blood to the farthest parts of the body.

As the walls of these vessels swell, there is less room for the blood to squeeze through. Blood keeps thudding into the swollen arteries, backs up and creates hypertension. In addition to swelling the arterioles, an excess of salt causes retention of body fluid, which results in more volume of blood and further raises the blood pressure. This in turn strains the heart.

John H. Laragh, M.D., professor of clinical medicine at Columbia University College of Physicians and Surgeons, when speaking on a WNBC-TV program in New York, said there is a striking fact about high blood pressure in "its close relationship to the amount of salt that a person eats.

"There is no doubt, both in experimental animals and in humans, the increased dietary salt consumption in various parts of the world is associated with much more high blood pressure and with a higher incidence of strokes. Conversely, there's no question about the beneficial effect of withholding salt from the diet of anyone with high blood pressure.

"While it is not altogether clear just how salt (sodium chloride) raises the blood pressure, it is believed that it creates a hydraulic effect by retaining fluid in the circuit, and this in turn tends *per se* to raise blood pressure." Or putting it simply, a large fluid volume demands more pressure to circulate.

Eors Bajusz, M.D., in *Nutritional Aspects of Cardiovascular Disease,* says that the body cannot tolerate salt excesses. "All mammals for millions of years have faced the desperate difficulty of conserving sodium, while only in the last 300 years have bodily processes begun to cope with the opposite problem, getting rid of the great excesses of sodium chloride contained in our modern diet."

Dr. Lewis K. Dahl, speaking before the McGovern Select Committee on Nutrition and Human Needs, explained that salt causes high blood pressure in test animals and could have the same effect in humans.

"The hypertension evoked in the test animal," Dr. Dahl says, "bears a striking resemblance to the common hypertension that afflicts man and runs from benign, slowly evolving elevation in pressure to high and rapidly fatal hypertension.

"Young animals are significantly more susceptible to the noxious effects of salt than are older animals. What's more, in studies with animals from a genetically hypertension-prone strain, even transient high salt intakes for as briefly as two to six weeks early in life, could induce permanent and sometimes fatal hypertension."

Dr. Dahl was able to induce hypertensive sta⁺

in test animals by feeding them commercial foods. But when other animals, who were also hypertension-prone were fed low-salt foods, they enjoyed normal blood pressure levels. He concluded that *added* sodium in processing, cooking or at the table was unhealthy, undesirable, and unnecessary.

It is highly possible that after a short non-salt period, you will find that you *prefer* food enhanced by the natural flavors of herbs and spices instead of blanketed by one taste—salt.

The following list offers seasonings available at health stores and shows how to add an exotic dash to everyday foods:

Allspice
Almond extract
Anise
Basil
Bay leaf
Caraway
Cardamom
Chili powder
Chives
Cinnamon
Cloves
Cocoa (not Dutch
    process)
Coconut
Coriander
Cumin
Curry powder
Dill
Fennel
Garlic
Ginger

Honey
Horseradish (not
    prepared)
Leeks
Lemon juice or extract
Mace
Maple syrup
Marjoram
Mint
Mustard, dry
Nutmeg
Onion juice
Orange extract
Oregano
Paprika
Parsley
Pepper, black, red or
    white
Peppermint extract
Peppers, fresh green
Pimento

Poppyseed
Poultry seasoning
Purslane
Rosemary
Saffron
Sage
Savory
Sesame

Sorrel
Tarragon
Thyme
Turmeric
Vanilla extract
Vinegar
Walnut extract

SODIUM-FREE BAKING POWDER

You may obtain this from some specialty food stores, or a pharmacist can prepare it from this formula (makes about 4 ounces):

Potassium bicarbonate	39.8 grams
Cornstarch	28.0 grams
Tartaric acid	7.5 grams
Potassium bi-tartrate	56.1 grams

Substitute 1½ teaspoons for 1 teaspoon of regular baking powder.

Above lists reprinted from N.R.C. Bulletin 325, "Sodium Restricted Diets."

Try These Seasonings With:

MEAT AND ALTERNATES

BEEF—dry mustard, marjoram, nutmeg, onion, sage, thyme, pepper, bay leaf, grape jelly, mushrooms, green peppers

PORK—onion, garlic, sage, applesauce, spiced apples

LAMB—mint, garlic, rosemary, curry, broiled pineapple rings

VEAL—bay leaf, ginger, marjoram, curry, currant jelly, spiced apricots, oregano

CHICKEN—paprika, mushrooms, thyme, sage, parsley, tarragon, cranberry sauce

FISH—dry mustard, paprika, curry, bay leaf, lemon juice, mushrooms, marjoram, green peppers

EGGS—pepper, green peppers, mushrooms, dry mustard, paprika, curry, onion, parsley

VEGETABLES

ASPARAGUS—lemon juice

BROCCOLI—lemon juice

BRUSSELS SPROUTS—marjoram

CABBAGE—mustard dressing, caraway seed, dill seed, unsalted butter with lemon and honey

CAULIFLOWER—nutmeg, thyme

CORN—green peppers, tomatoes

GREEN BEANS—marjoram, lemon juice, nutmeg, unsalted French dressing, dill seed

PEAS—mint, mushrooms, parsley, onion, rosemary

POTATOES—boiled, with parsley, unsalted butter, mace, chopped green peppers, onion

SQUASH—ginger, mace, nutmeg

SWEET POTATOES—candied or glazed with cinnamon or nutmeg; escalloped with apples, honey or orange slices

TOMATOES—basil, marjoram, onion, parsley

ZUCCHINI—oregano, garlic

SEVEN BASIC RULES FOR ENJOYING A SALT-FREE HEALTH PROGRAM

1. Ask your doctor to set your point limits for sodium, expressed in milligrams per day. He may

also want to give you other guidelines for enjoying healthier living to control blood pressure.

2. Plan ahead each day for the most delicious meals within your limits.

3. Keep a little score each day. This helps you stay within your goal and also helps you make certain you get the required nutrient values.

4. Get rid of your salt shaker! Avoid foods on the taboo list.

5. Be a label reader! When any label (food or drugs) contains these words, pass them by: salt, baking powder, brine, or ingredients including sodium, such as: monosodium glutamate, sodium benzoate, sodium bicarbonate, sodium sulfite, sodium hydroxide, sodium cyclamate.

6. Measure your foods. Use standard measuring cups and spoons in assorted sizes: cup, ½ cup, ⅓ cup, ¼ cup, 1 tablespoon, 1 teaspoon, ½ teaspoon, ¼ teaspoon.

7. Verify the sodium content of your local water supply. Call the Health Department and ask for a reading. This is important, if you have a water softener. You may be advised to drink and cook with a bottled water of low sodium content.

AVOID THESE HIGH-SODIUM FOODS

Artichokes	Dandelion Greens
Beet Greens	Kale
Beets	Mustard Greens
Carrots	Sauerkraut
Celery	Spinach
Chard	White Turnips

Whole Hominy

Bacon—Bacon Fat—
    Salt Pork
Bologna
Brains
Chipped Beef or
    Turkey
Corned Beef
Ham
Kidneys
Luncheon Meat
Sausage

Anchovies
Canned Tuna or
    Salmon
Caviar
Herring
Salted Nuts—Pretzels—
    Popcorn—Potato
    Chips—Corn Chips
Sardines
Shell Fish (Shrimp,
    Lobster, Oyster,
    Crabs, Scallops)

Canned Vegetables or
    Juices—unless special
    dietetic-low-sodium
    pack
Frozen Vegetables if
    processed with salt

Olives—Pickles—Relishes
Party Spreads and Dips

Ice Cream—Sherbet

Baking Powder
Baking Soda
Monosodium Glutamate

Commercial Salad
    Dressings or
    Mayonnaise

Low calorie soft
    drinks

Commercial Bouillon
    (cubes or powders)
Commercial Gelatin
    Dessert
Molasses

Pudding Mixes
Rennet Tablets

Catsup
Celery Leaves
Celery Salt
Celery Seed
Chili Sauce
Garlic Salt
Meat Sauces
Onion Salt
Prepared Mustard
Sodium Cyclamate
Soy Sauce
Water—if over 20
    milligrams per quart
Worcestershire Sauce

HELPFUL HINTS FOR SEASONING FOODS WITHOUT SALT

Because you have been using more salt than you really need, your taste buds want a tang of something exciting. Here are some ways to help you enjoy the flavor of natural foods, without salt:

*Use lemon and lime wedges. These tart fruits are just about sodium-free and can be used freely. As a salt substitute, try a squeeze of lemon or lime juice. You'll enjoy a fragrant, sharp flavor that makes up for the absence of salt.

*Adventure into the world of sodium-free herbs and spices. They add a varied interest to food. Try them individually or experiment with combinations for new flavor thrills.

*Avoid salt in cooking and at your table.

*Use unsalted butter or margarine.

*Most canned vegetables and soups are high in sodium. Read the labels.

*Many breakfast foods are high in sodium. Many others are low. Again, read the label.

*Homemade salad dressings made with vegetable oil, vinegar and spices contain little sodium, but commercial mayonnaise and commercial dressings may be high in sodium. Check the label.

*Most fresh meat and poultry products are low in sodium. But processed meats—ham, bacon, sausage, frankfurters and so on, are high in sodium and should be avoided.

*Similarly, *fresh* fish is rather low in sodium but processed fish may have salt added. The label will tell all.

*Use coffee substitutes and herbal teas. Use lemon and honey. Milk or cream may be added, if doctor-approved.

GUIDE TO APPROXIMATE MEASURES

(**Metric to U.S. common measures**)

Since you'll be reading different labels, you'll want to understand them. Here is a check list:

1 gram = 1000 milligrams
1 oz. = 30 grams
3.5 oz. = 100 grams
1 cup = 16 tablespoons
½ cup = 8 tablespoons
1 tablespoon = 3 teaspoons

Examples (based on average serving size):

One cup of milk equals 244 grams and contains 122 milligrams of sodium

One medium potato equals 150 grams and contains 4 milligrams of sodium

One tablespoon butter equals 30 grams and contains 3 milligrams of sodium

One vegetable serving equals 100 grams and usually contains 9 milligrams of sodium

Five ounces beef equals 120 grams and contains 104 milligrams of sodium

One serving citrus fruit equals 100 grams and contains 1 milligram of sodium

Use the following convenient chart as a guide when you plan your week's menu, in cooperation with your family doctor.

SODIUM COUNTER

This chart represents the number of milligrams of sodium in every 100 grams of the listed food or beverage. Since one-half cup of milk weighs approximately 122 grams and contains 61 milligrams of sodium, it is clear that the sodium content in even a small quantity can be substantial. The chart is designed to help you plan complete daily and weekly menus with reduced sodium and high nutritional value.

MEATS

Bacon, fried	2400
Beef, corned	1300
Beef, lean	70
Chicken, light meat	65
Chicken, dark meat	90
Duck	85
Frankfurters	1100
Ham	1100
Lamb, lean	90
Liver	130
Pork, lean	55
Sausage, pork	740
Turkey, white meat	40
Turkey, dark meat	92
Veal, lean	100

FISH

Clams, raw	180
Cod	60
Crab, canned	1000
Flounder	68
Lobster	250
Oysters	73
Salmon, canned	540
Shrimp	140
Tuna, canned	800

SNACKS

Candy, caramels	208
Milk Chocolate	86
Gum Drops	41
Candy, bars	200
Ice Cream	90
Cookies	163
Potato Chips	340
Pretzels	1700
Peanuts, salted	460
Cashews, salted	200

DAIRY PRODUCTS

Butter, salted	1000
Butter, sweet	880
Butter, unsalted	10
Cheese	700
Cheese, cottage	290
Cheese, process	1500
Eggs, whole	130
Margarine	1100
Milk	50

BREADS, CEREALS, OTHERS

Bread, rye & wheat	600

Bread, white	511
Bread, white enriched	500
Corn Flakes	660
Oats	1
Crackers, soda	1100
Crackers, graham	710
Macaroni, plain	5
Rice	12
Noodles, egg	10
Spaghetti	5

BEVERAGES

Beer, Wine	7
Orange juice	1
Coffee	2
Root Beer	8
Grape Soda	23
Soft Drinks	7
Tea	4

VEGETABLES

Artichoke	43
Asparagus, fresh	3
Asparagus, canned	410
Avocado	3
Beans, fresh green	1
Beans, canned green	410
Beans, fresh lima	1
Beans, canned lima	310
Beans, canned baked	591
Beets, fresh	60
Beets, canned	36
Broccoli	15
Brussels Sprouts	12
Cabbage	15
Carrots, fresh	50
Carrots, canned	280
Cauliflower	20
Celery	100
Corn, fresh	1
Corn, canned	200
Cucumbers	5
Lettuce	3
Olives, green	2400
Onions	1
Peas, fresh	2
Peas, canned	270
Potatoes	3
Radishes	15
Spinach, fresh	75
Spinach, canned	320
Tomatoes, fresh	3
Tomatoes, canned	18
Sauerkraut, canned	650

FRUITS

Apples	1
Apricots, fresh	1
Apricots, canned	4
Bananas	1
Blackberries	1
Cantaloupe	13
Cherries	2
Dates	1

Fruit Cocktail	9	Pineapple	1
Grapes	2	Plums, fresh	1
Grapefruit	2	Strawberries	1
Oranges	1	Watermelon	1
Peaches, fresh	1		
Peaches, canned	2		
Pears, fresh	2		
Pears, canned	2		

Compiled from a report of the Food and Nutrition Board, National Academy of Science, National Research Council.

HANDY GUIDE TO REDUCED SODIUM MENU PLANNING

You want to enjoy a healthy and flavorful diet. You can do this *without* salt. Simply be aware of what foods have high sodium content. It's more a matter of rethinking some of your buying habits, preparing fresh foods and using fewer mass-market packaged and processed foods.

Sodium is an element that is required by your body. Most foods contain sodium either naturally or through processing. Sodium is NOT salt. Salt is sodium chloride, a chemical flavoring added to commercial foods. Everyday foods contain *natural* sodium but you may want to cut down on some of these if your doctor approves and if he says you have high blood pressure.

Almost all foods have some natural sodium, but some contain only a very small amount. For example, fresh and canned fruits contain very little sodium while meats and dairy products contain more. All the food you eat or drink adds to the total amount of sodium in your daily diet. And when you add salt as a seasoning, you are likely to double that daily amount. Eliminate the salt shaker and you are off to a healthy start.

WHERE DO YOU BEGIN?

You begin by sitting down with your sodium chart and planning complete menus for the week. Advanced planning is essential if you are to cut down on salt consumption. If you go to the grocery store without a prepared list, you will be at a loss. Eventually, you will be so familiar with low-sodium foods that you will instinctively pick them off the shelf. But until you feel comfortable in knowing relative sodium amounts, it is better to plan ahead. When you make your list and when you go shopping, *use this book*. The charts and suggestions are instant computers to help you plan a low-salt eating program.

Remember, you do not have to learn any new way to cook. You just have to be aware of sodium content in your menu planning. One safe way is to prepare more foods from scratch, so that you know and can measure every ingredient. Another is to read carefully the content labels on prepared foods. You'll find, for example, that frozen vegetables have *little* sodium, while canned vegetables generally contain *added* sodium. You and your family will enjoy food just as much and find the flavor as appealing as that of meals high in sodium. It is a simple effective way to enjoy better health.

LOW-SALT MEATS

Different kinds of meats vary significantly in sodium content. Lean beef, veal and lamb are fairly low. So are chicken and turkey. Processed meats, such as sausage, frankfurters, bologna and lunch meats are high. Canned meat, fish or poultry generally have added salt. Smoked meats are always high and so are ham, pork, bacon and chipped and corned beef.

Meat may be broiled, baked or boiled. The cooking process doesn't usually add to the sodium content. Cooking oils contain essentially no sodium.

LOW-SALT FISH

Fresh fish fillets, whether fresh water or ocean, are low in sodium and can be served often. The sodium content goes up in canned fish. Shellfish are high in sodium, and salted or smoked fish are higher still. Be aware that anchovies and caviar are also very high in sodium count.

LOW-SALT VEGETABLES

Most fresh or frozen vegetables are not only nutritionally sound but relatively low in sodium. Since salt is added during processing, many canned vegetables have somewhat higher sodium content. Artichokes, carrots, celery and spinach are slightly higher than other vegetables.

LOW-SALT FRUITS

Fruits in any form—fresh, frozen, dried or canned—are low in sodium content and may be used freely in your menu planning. Try out your creativity and find new exciting ways to serve fresh or cooked fruit. There's no better dessert for you and your family.

LOW-SALT DAIRY PRODUCTS

Almost all dairy products are relatively high in sodium. Milk and cottage cheese are moderately high, other kinds of cheeses can be quite high. So dairy products do vary. But since we need a daily intake of proteins, they should not be eliminated from the diet. Use yogurt, too.

LOW-SALT BREADS, CEREALS

With few exceptions, *natural* cereals are good for you and contain little sodium. Some ready-to-serve and enriched cereals have added sodium. *Read the label!* Barley, cracked wheat, puffed wheat, shredded wheat, cream of wheat, oatmeal, grits, brown rice and cornmeal are usually low in sodium. Breads are moderately high in sodium. Find low-salt breads and bread products such as muffins, biscuits, rolls. If the product is low-salt or salt-free, it usually says so on the label.

LOW-SALT CONDIMENTS, SPICES

Many traditional condiments—ketchup, mustard, chili sauce, relishes, pickles—have high sodium content. So do barbecue sauce, soy sauce, Worcestershire sauce, bouillon cubes and canned sauces. You will do well to prepare your own sauce with an equal mixture of oil and apple cider vinegar with a bit of honey and some herbs. Salt-free spices are available and such products will tell you they have "no salt" on the label.

Health stores stock "dietetic foods" prepared with no added salt or they may be entirely sodium-free. A variety of such foods is available for your eating pleasure.

ELEVEN COMPOUNDS TO AVOID

Most foods contain some sodium, either because it is naturally present or because it has been added in one form or another. The American Heart Association says, "Sodium that is combined with another chemical element is frequently added to foods as they are processed or prepared. These sodium combinations—or compounds as they are called—can be recognized on food labels because they always contain the word *sodium* or *soda*. (The two words are often used interchangeably; for example, sodium bicarbonate or bicarbonate of soda.) Sometimes, you may see the chemist's symbol for sodium, *Na*. Watch for these compounds. Keep away from them." The Association offers this blacklist to help a salt-free diet:

1. *Salt* (sodium chloride)—used in cooking or at the table, and in canning and processing.
2. *Baking powder*—used to leaven quick breads and cakes.
3. *Baking soda* (sodium bicarbonate)—used to leaven breads and cakes; sometimes added to vegetables in cooking or used as an "alkalizer" for indigestion.
4. *Brine* (table salt and water)—used in processing foods to inhibit growth of bacteria; in cleaning or blanching vegetables and fruits; in freezing and canning certain foods; and for flavor, as in corned beef, pickles, sauerkraut.
5. *Di-sodium phosphate*—present in some quick-cooking cereals and processed cheeses.

6. *Monosodium glutamate* (sold under several brand names for home use)—used to enhance food flavor, especially in restaurant and hotel cooking and in some packaged, canned and frozen foods.
7. *Sodium alginate*—used in many chocolate milks and ice creams for smooth texture.
8. *Sodium benzoate*—used as a preservative in many condiments, such as relishes, sauces and salad dressings.
9. *Sodium hydroxide*—used in food processing to soften and loosen skins of ripe olives, hominy and some fruits and vegetables. It is also used in preparing Dutch process cocoa and chocolate.
10. *Sodium propionate*—used in pasteurized cheeses and in some breads and cakes to inhibit mold.
11. *Sodium sulfite*—used to bleach certain fruits for artificial color, such as maraschino cherries and glazed or crystallized fruit; also used as a preservative in some dried fruit, such as prunes. Read the label before you buy. Select sun-dried fruits.

About medicines. Some of these contain sodium. Always check with your doctor before you use any unprescribed medicine, even a headache remedy. The American Heart Association lists some medicines that may contain sodium:

"Alkalizers" for indigestion (such as bicarbonate of soda, rhubarb and soda)
> Antibiotics
> Cough medicines
> Laxatives
> Pain relievers
> Sedatives

Tooth pastes, tooth powders and mouth washes may also contain large amounts of sodium. If you don't swallow tooth paste, you don't need to worry. Just be sure to rinse well with water after brushing your teeth or after using a mouth wash.

A salt-free diet can contribute to healthy arteries and a long lifetime free of hypertension.

CHAPTER FOUR

THE BENEFITS OF A SUGAR-FREE DIET

Sugar in prepared and processed foods, sugar used in cooking and on the table, sugar used as a sweetener for beverages, is a contributing cause to hypertension. Many doctors now feel that white sugar and its cousin, white flour, are more responsible for high cholesterol and high blood pressure than are saturated fats.

Excessive refined sugar intake triggers the emotionally upsetting problem of hypoglycemia, or low blood sugar. This condition occurs when the body has to metabolize an overabundance of sugar.

In hypoglycemics, the pancreas (the gland located behind the lower part of the stomach) has become too sensitive, too active. It must produce an excessive amount of insulin to metabolize the sugar. This causes body sugar, or *glucose,* which the body has made from eaten food, to be burned up rapidly.

The resulting imbalance of hormones sets off an unhealthy chain reaction. The brain cells depend wholly on blood sugar for nourishment and are the first to suffer from this disorder. Nervous unrest and a form of hypertension with a related set of harmful reactions follow.

Essentially, excessive sugar intake causes an overworked pancreas brought on by over-stimulating the isles of Langerhans (the insulin-producing cells in the pancreas). Symptoms include hypertension with varying bouts of energy and tiredness, poor ability to concentrate, irregular appetite, anxiety, obesity, depression, muscular tension, restlessness, poor coordination, underachievement, speech difficulty, convulsions and more serious forms of mental illness.

The effect of hypoglycemia on the nerve tissues creates the erratic and nervous temperament connected with high blood pressure.

It is erroneously believed that eating sugar is a quick way to energy. Actually, eating food containing refined sugar or starch (which is quickly changed into sugar), causes body imbalance. The mechanism in the pancreas for handling sugar is either triggered too rapidly or is delayed and then set into action too rapidly. In the first case, the blood sugar shows little or no rise following the eating of sugar. In the second case, the blood sugar rises abnormally high and than abnormally low.

It is this see-saw, up-and-down insulin yank that leads to erratic and disturbed emotional temperament. Untreated, it can elevate the blood pressure, causing continued, unrelieved hypertension.

You may say you don't eat any sugar. But if you read the following chart, you will discover the amount of sugar in some processed foods that many people eat daily.

Food item	Size portion	Approximate sugar content in teaspoonfuls of granulated sugar
BEVERAGES		
COLA DRINKS	1 (6 oz. bottle or glass)	3½
CORDIALS	1 (¾ oz. glass)	1½
GINGER ALE	6 oz.	5
HI-BALL	1 (6 oz. glass)	2½
ORANGEADE	1 (8 oz. glass)	5
ROOT BEER	1 (10 oz. bottle)	4½
SEVEN-UP	1 (6 oz. bottle or glass)	3¾
SODA POP	1 (8 oz. bottle)	5
SWEET CIDER	1 cup	6
WHISKEY SOUR	1 (3 oz. glass)	1½
CAKES & COOKIES		
ANGEL FOOD	1 (4 oz. piece)	7
APPLE SAUCE CAKE	1 (4 oz. piece)	5½
BANANA CAKE	1 (2 oz. piece)	2
CHEESE CAKE	1 (4 oz. piece)	2
CHOCOLATE CAKE (Plain)	1 (4 oz. piece)	6
CHOCOLATE CAKE (Iced)	1 (4 oz. piece)	10
COFFEE CAKE	1 (4 oz. piece)	4½
CUP CAKE (Iced)	1	6
FRUIT CAKE	1 (4 oz. piece)	5
JELLY-ROLL	1 (2 oz. piece)	2½
ORANGE CAKE	1 (4 oz. piece)	4
POUND CAKE	1 (4 oz. piece)	5
SPONGE CAKE	1 (1 oz. piece)	2
STRAWBERRY SHORTCAKE	1 serving	4

The Benefits of a Sugar-free Diet

Food item	Size portion	Approximate sugar content in teaspoonfuls of granulated sugar
BROWNIES (Unfrosted)	1 (¾ oz.)	3
CHOCOLATE COOKIES	1	1½
FIG NEWTONS	1	5
GINGER SNAPS	1	3
MACAROONS	1	6
NUT COOKIES	1	1½
OATMEAL COOKIES	1	2
SUGAR COOKIES	1	1½
CHOCOLATE ECLAIR	1	7
CREAM PUFF	1	2
DONUT (Plain)	1	3
DONUT (Glazed)	1	6
SNAIL	1 (4 oz. piece)	4½

CANDIES

AVERAGE MILK CHOCOLATE BAR (example: Hershey bar)	1 (1½ oz.)	2½
CHEWING GUM	1 stick	½
CHOCOLATE CREAM	1 piece	2
BUTTERSCOTCH CHEW	1 piece	1
CHOCOLATE MINTS	1 piece	2
FUDGE	1 oz. square	4½
GUM DROP	1	2
HARD CANDY	4 oz.	20
LIFESAVERS	1	⅓
PEANUT BRITTLE	1 oz.	3½

CANNED FRUITS & JUICES

CANNED APPRICOTS	4 halves and 1 Tbsp. syrup	3½
CANNED FRUIT JUICES (Sweetened)	½ cup	2

Food item	Size portion	Approximate sugar content in teaspoonfuls of granulated sugar
CANNED PEACHES	2 halves and 1 Tbsp. syrup	3½
FRUIT SALAD	½ cup	3½
FRUIT SYRUP	2 Tbsp.	2½
STEWED FRUITS	½ cup	2

DAIRY PRODUCTS

ICE CREAM	⅓ pt. (3½ oz.)	3½
ICE CREAM BAR	1	1–7 depending on size
ICE CREAM CONE	1	3½
ICE CREAM SODA	1	5
ICE CREAM SUNDAE	1	7
MALTED MILK SHAKE	1 (10 oz. glass)	5

JAMS & JELLIES

APPLE BUTTER	1 Tbsp.	1
JELLY	1 Tbsp.	4–6
ORANGE MARMALADE	1 Tbsp.	4–6
PEACH BUTTER	1 Tbsp.	1
STRAWBERRY JAM	1 Tbsp.	4

DESSERTS, MISCELLANEOUS

APPLE COBBLER	½ cup	3
BLUEBERRY COBBLER	½ cup	3
CUSTARD	½ cup	2
FRENCH PASTRY	1 (4 oz. piece)	5
JELLO	½ cup	4½
APPLE PIE	1 slice (average)	7
APRICOT PIE	1 slice	7
BERRY PIE	1 slice	10
BUTTERSCOTCH PIE	1 slice	4
CHERRY PIE	1 slice	10

The Benefits of a Sugar-free Diet

Food item	Size portion	Approximate sugar content in teaspoonfuls of granulated sugar
CREAM PIE	1 slice	4
LEMON PIE	1 slice	7
MINCEMEAT PIE	1 slice	4
PEACH PIE	1 slice	7
PRUNE PIE	1 slice	6
PUMPKIN PIE	1 slice	5
RHUBARB PIE	1 slice	4
BANANA PUDDING	½ cup	2
BREAD PUDDING	½ cup	1½
CHOCOLATE PUDDING	½ cup	4
CORNSTARCH PUDDING	½ cup	2½
DATE PUDDING	½ cup	7
FIG PUDDING	½ cup	7
GRAPENUT PUDDING	½ cup	2
PLUM PUDDING	½ cup	4
RICE PUDDING	½ cup	5
TAPIOCA PUDDING	½ cup	3
BERRY TART	1	10
BLANC-MANGE	½ cup	5
BROWN BETTY	½ cup	3
PLAIN PASTRY	1 (4 oz. piece)	3
SHERBET	½ cup	9

SYRUPS, SUGARS & ICINGS

Food item	Size portion	Approximate sugar content in teaspoonfuls of granulated sugar
BROWN SUGAR	1 Tbsp.	3 (actual sugar content)
CHOCOLATE ICING	1 oz.	5
CHOCOLATE SAUCE	1 Tbsp.	3½
CORN SYRUP	1 Tbsp.	3 (actual sugar content)
GRANULATED SUGAR	1 Tbsp.	3 (actual sugar content)
HONEY	1 Tbsp.	3 (actual sugar content)

Food item	Size portion	Approximate sugar content in teaspoonfuls of granulated sugar
KARO SYRUP	1 Tbsp.	3 (actual sugar content)
MAPLE SUGAR	1 Tbsp.	5 (actual sugar content)
MOLASSES	1 Tbsp.	3½ (actual sugar content)
WHITE ICING	1 oz.	5

Source: American Foundation for Medical Dental Science Inc.: Dr. Michael J. Walsh.

HYPERTENSIVE REACTIONS TRACED TO HYPOGLYCEMIA

The hormonal imbalance of hypoglycemia often triggers hypertensive reactions. Many nervous persons are victims of sugar indulgence. Sugar-holics are vulnerable to emotional ailments. Harry H. Salzer, M.D., in the *Ohio State Medical Technical Bulletin,* cites three types of hypertensive-emotional ailments traced to excessive sugar indulgence:

1. *Psychiatric symptoms:* Depression, insomnia, anxiety, irritability, lack of concentration, crying spells, phobias, forgetfulness, confusion, antisocial behavior and even suicidal tendencies
2. *Neurological symptoms:* Headaches, dizziness, trembling, numbness, blurred vision, staggering, fainting or blackouts, muscular twitching
3. *Intensive somatic symptoms:* Exhaustion, fatigue, bloating, abdominal spasms, muscle and joint pains, backaches, muscle cramps, colitis and convulsions

Dr. Salzer says that hypoglycemia can duplicate many neuro-psychiatric disorders. He says some

cases have been incorrectly diagnosed as schizophrenia, manic-depression and psychotic or psycho-
pathic personality development. But when patients
were placed on a high-protein, low-sugar, low-car-
bohydrate food plan, blood pressure returned to
acceptable limits and improvement continued.

DR. SEALE HARRIS'S TWO-WEEK PLAN
TO LOWER HYPERTENSION

This is often called the *Harris Diet*, because it
was developed by Seale Harris, M.D., the pioneer-
discoverer of hypoglycemia; it is reportedly able to
help stabilize the blood pressure at a lower rate.

YOU MUST ABSOLUTELY AVOID:

1. Sugar, candy, cake, pie, pastries, sweet custards,
   puddings, ice cream and all other sweets
2. Potatoes, white rice, grapes, raisins, plums, figs,
   dates and bananas
3. Spaghetti, macaroni and noodles
4. Caffeine—ordinary coffee, tea and cola drinks,
   including the low-calorie cola drinks
5. All wines, cocktails, beer and cordials

YOU ARE ALLOWED:

1. Asparagus, broccoli, brussels sprouts, cabbage,
   cauliflower, carrots, celery, corn, cucumbers,
   eggplant, lima beans, onions, peas, radishes, sauerkraut, squash, stringbeans, turnips, tomatoes
2. Apples, apricots, berries, grapefruit, melon,
   oranges, peaches, pears, pineapple, tangerines
   (Dr. Harris says that fruits may be eaten either
cooked or raw but NO sugar may be used, either

added or in canned fruits. If you buy sugar-packed canned fruit, then rinse it twice with free flowing water; let stand overnight in water to help remove the sugar. Health stores sell sugar-free canned fruits.)

3. Lettuce, mushrooms and nuts may be taken as often as needed, as a snack at any time. *But—* one-half ounce or a handful of nuts at one time and no more

4. Any unsweetened fruit or vegetable juice, except grape or prune juice may be taken

5. Weak tea, decaffeinated coffee or coffee substitutes are acceptable beverages. NO sweetening with sugar

6. Fruit desserts without sugar; also, low-calorie and sugar-free gelatin desserts are acceptable

HERE IS THE TWO-WEEK FOOD PLAN

Dr. Seale Harris developed this diet for his hypertensive patients. Since any corrective food program is individual, you are advised to obtain a personally prescribed diet from your physician. This special Harris plan for helping the control of high blood pressure is offered as a guide:

On arising: Medium orange or four ounces of juice or half grapefruit

Breakfast: Fruit or four ounces of juice; one egg, one slice only of bread with butter, beverage

Two hours after breakfast: Four ounces of juice

Lunch: Fish, cheese, meat or eggs, salad, large serving of lettuce, tomato or apple salad with mayonnaise or French dressing, vegetables if desired, only one slice of any bread or toast, dessert, beverage

Three hours after lunch: Four ounces of milk

Dinner: Soup, if desired (not thickened), vegetable, liberal portion of meat, fish or poultry, one slice of bread, dessert, beverage

Two-three hours after dinner: Four ounces of milk

Every two hours until bedtime: Four ounces of milk or a handful of nuts

This food plan helps the hormonal system, lessens the risk of hypoglycemia and promotes a more healthful blood pressure level.

Psychiatrist Juan Carlos DeTata, M.D., according to his medical paper entitled, *Research On Relative Hypoglycemic Syndrome,* treats hypertensive patients at a special health center by using prescribed sugar-free nutritional therapy. Dr. DeTata writes of the wonderful results:

"We have at this health clinic carried out a very simple research consisting of twenty-three patients who came for outpatient hypertensive treatment in which we suspected the presence of relative hypoglycemic syndrome.

"We utilized a very similar diet to the so-called Harris Diet and we were able to bring about a tremendous emotional improvement in those hypertensive patients who cooperated with the diet.

"It is also interesting to note that the local people's diet is mostly starchy, consisting of rice and some vegetable products and they have tremendous difficulty in following a high-protein diet. Also, they are reluctant to abandon coffee. However, in the few cases that did follow our diet, they improved wonderfully!

"Increased ingestion of *calcium* to improve their concomitant hypocalcemia was also recommended . . . We certainly insist that every patient with emotional upset try to discover if he is not suffering concomitantly from relative hypoglycemia."

THE TINTERA PROGRAM FOR HYPERTENSIVES

The well-known John W. Tintera, M.D., in the *New York State Journal of Medicine,* states that eight out of ten hypertensive persons may be victims of hypoglycemia. He prepared a program intended to control and relieve hypoglycemia and hypertension:

FOODS ALLOWED:

> All meats, fish
> Dairy products (eggs, milk, butter and cheese. Also recommended—1 pint to one quart of acidophilus milk daily). Milk between meals; milk, cheese before retiring
> All vegetables and fruits not listed below
> Nuts as in-between meal snacks in moderation
> Peanut butter
> Sanka, weak tea and sugar-free sodas
> Soybeans and soybean products

FOODS TO AVOID:

> Potatoes, corn, macaroni, spaghetti, rice
> Pie, cake, pastries, sugar, candies
> Dates and raisins
> Cola and other sweet soft drinks
> Coffee and strong tea
> All hot and cold cereals (except occasionally oatmeal)
> Alcoholic beverages, narcotics and drugs which act as stimulant or depressant

Dr. Tintera's diet essentially consists of the elimination of rapidly absorbed carbohydrates in order to obviate the hormonal reaction of rapidly rising blood sugar and its subsequent fall. By leveling this up-down yank, the nervous system is soothed. There is a gradual stabilization of hypertension as natural tranquility is restored.

THE PROGRAM THAT SAVED A HYPERTENSIVE

In the *Journal of Schizophrenia*, Robert L. Meiers, M.D., writes of his use of nutrition to treat a California woman. She had had severe hypertension for years. She was also under severe pressure. She smoked heavily. She consumed endless amounts of coffee. She ate a high-starch, high-sugar diet. The more tense, tired and depressed she became, the more she reached for artificial stimulants.

When examined by the doctor, she was found to have hypoglycemia as well as hypertension. She was put on a low-starch, low-sugar diet with considerable protein and moderate fat. No coffee. No cigarettes. No alcohol.

She began to recover. Tensions melted slowly. Dr. Meiers then gave her large amounts of niacin and vitamin C. She also started to take brewer's yeast daily. She "noticed a marked increase in her energy level in one week." Soon she was able to meet her obligations, adjust to the world and get a good job.

Because emotional distress is often traced to hypertension, B-complex vitamins are frequently advised in treatment. Dr. Meiers says that one cause for improvement in hypertension is the use of brewer's yeast since, as he writes, "no commercial vitamin preparation contains all the known B-complex vitamins. Also, there probably are B-complex factors not yet identified and about the only natural sources of all the B-complex vitamins are liver, brewer's yeast and wheat germ."

A typical hypoglycemia program for hypertensives as prescribed by Dr. Meiers includes the following:

First month: A diet to treat low blood sugar. Eliminate any stimulants such as coffee, pep pills, alcohol and smoking. He gives from 3000 to 4000 milligrams of vitamin C daily to his patients.

Second month: Large doses of niacin, the B^3 vitamin, while the patient follows the same program as the first month.

Third month: Vitamin-mineral supplementation in addition to the above.

Fourth month: Increased B-complex vitamins, in addition to the above.

This program is reportedly helpful in soothing hypertension, regulating blood pressure and lessening the symptoms of hypoglycemia.

Sugar is a non-food, a pure carbohydrate that causes irregularity of the nervous system. It sops up the vitamin B-complex group in order to be metabolized. These vitamins are needed to nourish the nervous system. A deficiency can cause hypertension. The sugar molecule is something like: $C_n H_2N O_n$ (Carbon, hydrogen, oxygen). It has no nutrients. It is water-soluble and rushes into the bloodstream. It disrupts normal health patterns and blood pressure.

By using healthful foods and eliminating refined carbohydrates from your diet, you will help your nervous system and be working towards the maintenance of normal blood pressure.

CHAPTER FIVE

THE CAFFEINE-FREE WAY

CAFFEINE CAUSES AN UNHEALTHY RISE IN blood pressure.

Soft drinks as well as coffee and tea, are prime sources of the hypertension-causing drug known as *caffeine*. It contributes to emotional stress and provokes blood pressure to violent fluctuations. Caffeine is an unhealthy substance and should be restricted.

By strict definition, caffeine is a crystallizable, slightly bitter, stimulating alkaloid found in the leaves and berries of the coffee plant. It is also chemically identified with the thein (alkaloid) found in tea leaves. Caffeine is found in almost all soft drinks such as the cola beverages.

Cola, botanically speaking, comes from a small genus of tropical African trees bearing a seed, the cola nut. When used in soft drinks, the caffeine in the cola nut affects blood pressure.

HOW CAFFEINE DISTURBS NERVE HEALTH

Bridges' *Dietetics For The Clinician* says, "Coffee and tea stimulate the nervous system, more especially the higher centers and may temporarily induce mental clarity, facilitating the reception of sensory impressions and the removal of the sense of fatigue."

Impairs sleep. "Definite impairment of sleep usually results from the consumption of an amount equivalent to 6 grains of caffeine (5 to 6 cups of tea or 3 to 4 cups of coffee). There may result a slight vaso-dilatation of the peripheral blood vessels. In the unaccustomed, the blood pressure rises slightly and then falls, the pulse is usually accelerated and a diuresis (promoted excretion of urine) is evident. Overindulgence may bring about frequent premature cardiac contractions. Habitual users of these beverages show little, if any, effect on the rate, force and output of the heart."

Influences respiratory health. "Tea and coffee directly stimulate the respiratory center and the respiratory rate increases. There is a slight increase in the basal metabolic rate reported by most observers." This also causes blood pressure variations.

Affects the central nervous system. The *British Pharmaceutical Code* reports, "Caffeine acts on the central nervous system, on muscle, including cardiac muscles, and on the kidneys.

"The action on the central nervous system is mainly on the higher centers and produces a condition of wakefulness and increased mental activity . . . With large doses of caffeine, the action extends from the physical areas to the motor area, the medulla and the (spinal) cord, and the patient becomes at first restless, and later may show convulsive movements."

Drs. Goodman and Gilman, in *The Pharmacological Basis of Therapeutics,* tell us, "Excitation of the central nervous system is usually followed by depression" after much caffeine intake through coffee, tea or cola drinks. The doctors say, "Insomnia, restlessness and excitement are the earliest symptoms and may progress to a mild delirium. Tachycardia (increased heartbeat) and extra systoles (irregular heart function) are frequent, and the respiration is quickened. The diuretic action of the drug (caffeine) may be prominent."

Dr. William T. Salter, professor of pharmacology, Yale University of Medicine, says, "The chief problem . . . is the possible chronic effect on the central nervous system . . . increased irritability, loss of sleep, palpitation of the heart, and even muscular tremors.

"Such effects are due to chronic mild intoxication with caffeine. Tea contains over twice as much caffeine as coffee, but as it is ordinarily brewed, there is approximately the same amount of caffeine present in the ordinary cup of tea as in a cup of coffee, i.e., 150 milligrams (one therapeutic dose). In both cases, the nervous effects are due primarily to caffeine. Certain widely used soft drinks . . . also contain as much caffeine as ordinary coffee."

Lloyd Rosenvold, M.D., in *Nutrition For Life,* alerts us, also, to the presence of caffeine in soft drinks. "Many soft drinks containing caffeine are sold on the market. Chief among these are the various 'cola' beverages, some of which have been found to contain as much as two-thirds to one and one-fourth grains of caffeine per cup or bottle. The deleterious effects on the body are very similar to those of coffee."

Drains nervous energy. J. Wayne McFarland, M.D., in *Better Living,* cautions: "Caffeine is a stimulant to nerves. Even though they need rest, caffeine makes people keep on working. Caffeine whips up muscles to keep moving when they are trying to relax. It makes the brain keep on working after it has begged for just a little respite. It aggravates nervous or overworked stomachs and gives one a sense of energy which the body does not have. It cuts into one's reserves and affects the heart.

"Whether taken in large or small quantities, its effects are always the same," says Dr. McFarland. "For many, it is only a little poison now and then. And though taken with meals, it is lacking in vitamins, minerals or food value of any kind. *It is still a drug.* And where do we find this caffeine? In coffee, tea and cola drinks."

Lowers blood sugar. J. DeWitt Fox, M.D., in *The Best Of Life And Health,* says: "caffeine also dissipates blood sugar by draining your reserve sugar from the liver. This is why you may get a temporary lift from a cup of coffee. But you know from experience that it isn't long before the letdown after your cup of coffee. This is because of lowered blood sugar."

Dr. Fox suggests, "For a refreshing beverage, try fruit juices—orange, pineapple, grape or lemonade."

Develops stimulant dependancy. Hypertension is closely related to the nervous system. Whatever disturbs the nervous system also causes variations in blood pressure. Coffee is such a disturbance, says Dr. Fox. "Coffee not only elevates stomach acidity to excessive levels but also strongly stimulates the central nervous system, speeds the heart, raises blood pressure. The 'wake up' cup of coffee, which is a must with so many, is an artificial stimulus to the nervous system, which soon calls for another.

"The midmorning letdown calls for a pick-me-up cup of coffee. Unfortunately, the taking of all stimulating drugs, of which caffeine as found in coffee is one, is followed by a period of depression. The letdown period calls for another cup of coffee and accounts for the powerful habit-forming properties of all caffeine-containing beverages.

"When one realizes that the average cup of coffee contains one and one-half to two grains of caffeine, the cumulative dose that Americans are taking each day is appalling. Were it not for the tolerance which is built up to this drug, as taken in the coffee cup, jangled nerves would never be able to stand the overwhelming shocks of such doses of caffeine."

Dr. Fox points out that the "dose of caffeine given to a patient in coma in cases of extreme emergency is seven and one-half grains—equivalent to four or five cups of coffee. The shock of such a dose often arouses a patient from deep stupor to consciousness, so violent is the reaction upon his brain cells. Yet millions of Americans daily jolt their brains into extreme irritability by taking a like amount of caffeine in coffee."

Flogs exhausted nerves. Dr. Fox then asks, "Now, what effect does coffee and caffeine have on the hypertensive person? Already a nervous, high-strung person, he winds up his clockspring even tighter when he drinks a nerve stimulant such as coffee. Coffee keys him up, makes him more tense. It runs up his blood pressure by constricting tiny blood vessels and urging his heart to beat faster and more forcefully. His stomach secretes more acid. He

75

runs the risk of developing an ulcer of the stomach.

"Coffeetime," says Dr. Fox, "considered by many as a relaxing rest period during a day's work, is really 'flogging time.' The brain and nerves are tired and ask for a rest. But instead of lying down and taking a few minutes of rest, or a cat nap, the coffee drinker flogs the nervous system by an artificial stimulus—caffeine—to work when it is fatigued.

"His brain and nerves are crying for a letup, but he gulps a cup of coffee, obliterates the danger signals, and drives recklessly on through red lights. Eventually, the nervous system becomes so tense and taut that, like a clock that is wound too tightly, the spring snaps, and the person has a nervous breakdown or develops various illnesses.

"It is this stimulative effect of coffee on which so many rely for late hours of study, work or driving. It is against all the laws of health to overtax our nervous energy to the point of fatigue, then flog ourselves to the utmost by taking stimulants. The person with stomach disorders must abstain from stimulants and irritants if he hopes for a cure," Dr. Fox concludes.

CAFFEINE IS A MOOD-CHANGING DRUG

Consumer Reports compares a cup of caffeine-containing coffee to a "drug-containing substance" which "exercises a mild but real effect on the state of the emotions." They say further that caffeine as well as other mood-changing drugs may even have a cumulative effect and cause reactions over a course of years. Perhaps many emotionally upset persons are victims of the prolonged use of caffeine in coffee, tea and cola drinks.

Some of the physio-neurological effects of caffeine in soft drinks upon the system are listed by Drs. A. C. Ivy and J. A. Roth in *Gastroenterology:*

Caffeine produces gastro-duodenal ulcers in animals when the drug is given in such a way as to keep the animals' stomachs absorbing caffeine continuously.

Caffeine moderately stimulates the flow of gastric juices.

Caffeine produces very definite changes in the blood vessels of animals; these are similar to changes produced by prolonged resentment, hostility and anxiety.

As we know, ulcerous conditions are augmented by nervous unrest and excessive flow of hydrochloric acid in the stomach. Caffeine appears to hasten this combination of nervous factors.

How much caffeine is there in cola drinks? According to *Let's Talk About Food,* published by the American Medical Association:

"Cola drinks, including 'diet colas' may contain up to 72 milligrams of caffeine per 12 ounces, or 6 milligrams per fluid ounce; the popular cola beverages contain approximately 3 to 4.6 milligrams of caffeine per fluid ounce. A 5-ounce cup of coffee, prepared from 15 to 17 grams of coffee grounds, contains about 18 milligrams of caffeine per fluid ounce (90 milligrams)."

So cola drinks may contain a substantial amount of caffeine. It would be well to eliminate such beverages. Switch to fresh fruits and vegetables and their juices. These are delicious and healthy for the nervous system and the blood pressure levels.

OBSERVATIONS ON CAFFEINE BY PHYSICIANS

Dr. Jean Bogert in *Nutrition And Physical Fitness:* caffeine-containing coffee quickens the respiration, intensifies the pulse, raises the blood pressure, stimulates the kidneys, excites the function of the brain and temporarily relieves fatigue or depression.

Dr. Max M. Rosenberg in the *Encyclopedia of Medical Self-Help:* caffeine-coffee should be avoided by anyone who has heart disease, angina, high blood pressure, stomach trouble, skin ailments, arthritis or liver trouble.

G. G. Duncan, M.D., in *Diseases of Metabolism:* caffeine causes an increase of 3 to 10 percent in the basic metabolic rate within the first hour after the beverage is taken.

In *Let's Talk About Food,* issued by the American Medical Association, these questions and answers appear:

Question: Several brands of coffee claim to have 97 percent of their caffeine removed. Is this possible, and, if so, how is the caffeine extracted from the coffee beans?

Answer: The most common procedure for decaffeinating coffee is to soften the coffee beans by steaming them under pressure. The caffeine is then extracted with alcohol, while the extracting solvents are driven out by resteaming. After treatment, the coffee beans are roasted, packed and sold like the standard coffee. Manufacturers have not yet been able to remove all the caffeine; their best efforts produce coffee containing about 0.05 percent caffeine, or about 3 percent of the original amount. Regular coffee contains from 1.5 percent to 1.9 percent caffeine.

Question: Are coffee, tea and cola beverages harmful because of their caffeine content?

Answer: Tolerance to caffeine varies widely among individuals. A normal person can tolerate the amount of caffeine in most beverages without apparent discomfort, but people with such illnesses as active peptic ulcers, hypertension and cardio-vascular as well as nervous system disorders usually must restrict their intake of caffeine-containing products because of the stimulating effect.

The caffeine in coffee, among other effects on the nervous system, can cause sleeplessness. A cup of tea of average strength contains approximately 12 to 15 milligrams per fluid ounce or 60 to 75 milligrams per cup.

Question: Does the method of preparation affect the caffeine content of coffee?

Answer: Yes! Drip and vacuum coffee contain the least amount of caffeine; percolated coffee contains slightly more caffeine than does drip coffee; boiled coffee contains more caffeine than either drip or percolated. The caffeine contained in a cup of instant coffee is high, but the amount of coffee used will determine the caffeine content of the beverage. Generally, the average cup contains about 1.5 to 2.5 grains of caffeine; but this, again, will depend upon the strength of the brew.

The former AMA president, Morris Fishbein, M.D., in his *Handy Home Medical Adviser:* "Coffee has long been used as a stimulating and pleasant drink. A cup of coffee made with a tablespoonful of coffee contains from one and one-half to three grains of caffeine, a drug which stimulates the nervous system. People who have used coffee regularly can get over-stimulated. Some people claim that coffee interferes with sleep. For them, coffees are available which have had the caffeine greatly reduced or well-nigh eliminated. Caffeine appears also in tea, and there are similar substances in cocoa."

"Caffeine," Dr. Fishbein says, "has a stimulating effect on the body as a whole and can increase the flow of urine. It stimulates the mind, also."

To sum up: caffeine is a drug that whips up the nervous system, and predisposes elevation of the blood pressure. Avoid coffee, tea and cola drinks. Switch to coffee substitutes such as dandelion root, Postum and other such products available at all health stores, or to herb teas that are free of caffeine. Enjoy fruit and vegetable juices in endless exciting combinations. This is a good way to be kind to your nervous system and to help control hypertension.

CHAPTER SIX

ENJOY A LOW-FAT DIET

SATURATED FATS, UNSATURATED FATS, CHOLES-terol—what's all the fuss about? Does a diet high in saturated fats raise the blood cholesterol level and cause constriction of the arteries, thereby forcing the heart to pound harder as the blood pressure increases? It is generally believed so. Saturated fats may predispose a condition of hypertension by intensifying the problem of atherosclerosis. Deposition of cholesterol in the artery wall will also provoke high blood pressure, as will increased cholesterol production in the liver. A wise course is to reduce an excessive amount of saturated fats in the diet.

Cholesterol controversy. Cholesterol is one of several fat-like substances present in all blood serum. The body makes its own cholesterol. It is a natural product of the body and an essential part of the diet. But certain fatty foods lend themselves to excess production of cholesterol. These should be controlled.

The typical American menu features heavily marbled meats, fat-laden beverages, snacks and desserts which load the diet with an excess of saturated fats and cholesterol as well. The amount of cholesterol in the food you eat influences the amount in your bloodstream. Many doctors think that this results in a tendency to hypertension, atherosclerosis and heart problems. However, there is a growing belief among scientists that refined carbohydrates— white sugar and white flour—in conjunction with saturated fats—are the culprits, particularly in incidents of coronary thrombosis. It can do no harm to correct the diet by emphasizing moderation in saturated fat intake and eliminating the refined carbohydrates.

FATS—SATURATED VS. UNSATURATED

Physicians know that it is possible to lower blood cholesterol levels by controlling the fats in the diet. Two kinds of dietary fat need to be distinguished: saturated fats vs. unsaturated fats.

Saturated fats are basically those found in dairy products, solid fats and meats; they tend to be more or less solid at room temperature.

Unsaturated fats are found in fish and most vegetable oils; they are usually liquid at room temperature. Many foods contain *both* saturated and unsaturated fats.

Monounsaturated fats, found in a few foods, do not affect cholesterol one way or the other.

A partial listing of common foods according to fat content follows:

CHOLESTEROL CONTENT OF SOME SELECTED FOODS

MEAT, FISH AND EGGS

	Cholesterol (mg)
Liver (3½-oz. serving)	300
Eggs (1 large)	275
Oysters (5 to 8)	200
Lobster (3½-oz. serving)	200
Shrimp (10 small)	125
Clams (5 to 10)	99
Veal (3½-oz. serving)	90
Pork (3½-oz. serving)	70
Beef (3½-oz. serving)	70
Lamb (3½-oz. serving)	70
Freshwater fish (3½-oz. serving)	70
Chicken (3½-oz. serving)	60

DAIRY FOODS

	Cholesterol (mg)
Whole milk (8-oz. glass)	27
American cheese (1 oz.)	25
Ice cream (¼ pint)	23–34
Heavy cream (1 tbsp.)	17
Creamed cottage cheese (½ cup)	14
Butter (1 pat)	12
Gouda cheese (1 oz.)	10
Yogurt (½ cup)	6
Half and half (1 tbsp.)	5
Skim milk (8-oz. glass)	1

Source: American Dairy Council

FOODS ACCORDING TO TYPES OF FATS*

Predominantly Saturated Fats	Predominantly Polyunsaturated Fats	Predominantly Monounsaturated Fats
Meat—beef, veal,**lamb, pork and their products such as cold cuts, sausages	Liquid vegetable oils*** corn, cottonseed, safflower, soybean	Olive oil Olives Avocados Cashew nuts
Eggs	Margarines containing substantial amounts of the above oils in liquid form	
Whole milk		
Whole milk cheese		
Cream, sweet and sour	Fish	
Ice cream	Mayonnaise, salad dressing	
Butter		
Some margarines	Nuts—walnuts, filberts, pecans, almonds, peanuts	
Lard		
Hydrogenated shortenings		
Chocolate	Peanut butter	
Coconut	Products made from or with the above	
Coconut oil		
Products made from or with the above, such as most cakes, pastry, cookies, gravy, sauces and many snack foods		

*Based on *How to Follow the Prudent Diet*, N.Y.C. Dept. of Health, 1969.

**Veal and poultry (chicken and turkey) are relatively low in total fat. Veal fat is predominantly saturated; chicken and turkey fat is more favorably distributed between polyunsaturated and saturated fat.

***Peanut oil is not polyunsaturated to the same degree as the other oils.

Getting enough cholesterol. Cholesterol is a normal constituent of blood and tissues, found in every body cell. Some of that cholesterol is synthesized by your body; some is supplied by your diet. The amount supplied by your diet varies greatly, depending upon the kinds and amounts of foods included. Ordinary diets are likely to supply 600 to 900 milligrams of cholesterol daily. A "low-cholesterol" diet usually provides about 300 milligrams of cholesterol daily, an amount believed adequate. But only your physician can confirm this for your specific situation.

Getting enough polyunsaturated fatty acids. These essential fatty acids are needed to help control cholesterol levels. They are usually oils and are most abundant in plant seeds and fish oils. The most important fatty acids are *linoleic acid* and *arachidonic acid.* In particular, you need linoleic acid. It is an essential nutrient. It must be supplied by food. Your body cannot make it. It is involved in the metabolism of cholesterol and has other beneficial functions that are evident but have not yet been clearly defined. You need these polyunsaturated essential fatty acids.

Food sources: Salad and cooking oils such as safflower, sunflower, corn, cottonseed, soybean, sesame or peanut. Use these oils for cooking and in salads for taste and health.

SUGGESTIONS FOR CONTROLLING CHOLESTEROL-CAUSED HYPERTENSION

The Inter-society Commission For Heart Disease Resources issued a report entitled, *Primary Prevention of the Atherosclerotic Disease* in which they offered the following recommendations for controlling cholesterol-caused hypertension. (They recommend that dietary habits be adjusted early in childhood, in order to reduce the risk of coronary heart disease later.)

Adjust caloric intake to maintain optimu weight.

Reduce fat intake so that fat supplies less than 35 percent of the total calories.

Maintain a daily intake of less than 10 percent of the total calories from saturated fat and less than 10 percent from polyunsaturated fats, with the remainder of fat supplied by monounsaturated fats.

Plan a daily intake of less than 300 milligrams of cholesterol.

Use all possible controls of hypertension including the elimination of cigarette smoking.

HOW TO CONTROL YOUR INTAKE OF CHOLESTEROL-RICH FOODS

The American Heart Association explains, "You may have to change some of your long-standing eating habits, but you won't have to give up all of your favorite dishes." They offer these suggestions:

Eat no more than three egg yolks a week, including eggs in cooking.

Limit your use of shellfish and organ meats.

In most of your meat meals for the week, use fish, chicken, turkey and veal; limit beef, lamb to five moderate-size portions per week.

Choose lean cuts of meat, trim visible fat, and discard the fat that cooks out of the meat.

Avoid deep fat frying; use cooking methods that help to remove fat—baking, boiling, broiling, roasting, stewing.

Restrict (or eliminate) your use of fatty "luncheon" and "variety" meats like sausages and salami.

Instead of butter and other cooking fats that are solid or completely hydrogenated, use liquid vegetable oils rich in polyunsaturated fats.

Instead of whole milk and cheeses made from whole milk and cream, use skimmed milk and skimmed milk cheeses.

CONTROL FAT INTAKE IN MEAT

Even lean meat has fat in it. Here are some ways to reduce the saturated fat in meat:

Use a rack to drain off the fat when broiling, roasting or baking. Instead of basting with drippings, keep meat moist by pouring fruit juice, tomato juice or bouillon over it.

Cook one day ahead: stews, boiled meat, soup stock, or other dishes in which fat cooks into the liquid. After the food has been refrigerated, the hardened fat can be removed from the top.

Make gravies after the fat has hardened and can be removed from the liquid.

Broil, rather than pan-fry meats such as hamburger, lamb chops, steak.

When a recipe calls for browning the meat first, try browning it under the broiler instead of in a pan.

ENJOY VEGETABLES THE HEALTHY WAY

Vegetables can be made delicious by the addition of herbs and spices; see the suggested combinations in Chapter Three.

Start with a small quantity of seasoning (⅛ to ½ teaspoon) then let your own and your family's taste be your guide. Chopped parsley and chives, sprinkled on just before serving, also enhance the flavor of many vegetables.

Try cooking vegetables in vegetable oil, adding a little water during cooking if needed. Use 1 to 2 teaspoons of oil for each serving. Place in a skillet with tight cover. Season. Steam over very low heat until vegetables are done.

HOW TO USE VEGETABLE OILS

Liquid vegetable oils or margarines high in polyunsaturates can be used in many ways in cooking. For example:

To brown lean meats, and to pan- or oven-fry fish and poultry

To saute onions and other vegetables for soup

In cream sauces and soups made with skimmed milk

In whipped or scalloped potatoes with skimmed milk added

For making hot breads, pie crust and cakes

For popping corn and making snacks

In casseroles made with dried peas or beans

In browning rice or with Spanish rice or curried rice

For pancakes or waffles

A SUBSTANCE THAT MAY CAUSE HIGH BLOOD PRESSURE

Found in large amounts in *shellfish*, the industrial pollutant *cadmium* may be dangerously raising blood pressure.

This is the testimony given by Dr. H. Mitchell Perry, Jr., before Senator Philip Hart's (D.-Mich.) environmental subcommittee hearings on fish inspection. The professor from Washington University, St. Louis, stressed that the toxic metal is also being used increasingly in industrial plating, galvanizing and battery-making, and that the strong suspicion of its link with an increased incidence of high blood pressure "warrants an attempt to lower the cadmium exposure of the American people."

Test studies. In feeding studies made on animals,

Dr. Perry reported that nearly all of them given cadmium in their diet developed serious hypertension (high blood pressure) within three months. At the same time, control animals (fed and treated in the same way but without cadmium) maintained normal pressure.

Dr. Perry pointed out that cadmium is markedly concentrated in the kidney—the organ which is believed to be implicated in the pathogenesis (disease-causing) of hypertension. In body chemistry, Dr. Perry said, cadmium is bound to an unusual protein that binds both cadmium and the essential nutritive trace metal, zinc.

Doctors have also pointed to zinc's role in maintaining normal blood pressure and cited cadmium's harmful effect in "crowding out" the needed zinc.

Dr. Perry told the Senate committee, "Although at present there is no positive evidence that cadmium accumulation from long-term, low-level exposure is harmful," he emphasized that "its potential damage to the body may be irreversible."

It may be wise to eliminate shellfish from your food program. Choose other kinds of fish instead.

TWO FOOD ADDITIVES THAT RAISE
BLOOD PRESSURE

Two food additives, *nitrates* and *nitrites* are culprits in elevated pressure. These chemicals are usually found in smoked fish, processed meats, hot dogs, luncheon meats, cured hams, corned beef. They are also found in some water supplies. They preserve foods, but are harmful to the system. They are particularly involved in problems concerning cancer, heart trouble and hypertension.

Dr. William E. Morton, professor of Public health and preventive medicine at the University of Oregon Medical School, gave a report on this problem before the American Public Health Association annual meeting. Dr. Morton said that there was a surprisingly high incidence of hypertension and death from that ailment in a region where there is a high nitrate pollution in the drinking water.

Dr. Morton tells of findings to support his theory. "Chronic cardiovascular toxic effects among workers exposed to organic nitrates in industry include: elevated diastolic blood pressure, lowered pulse pressure, and increased risk of angina pectoris and/ or sudden death. In Pennsylvania, male workers aged 20–54 years have been reported to have a coronary artery disease mortality rate about 15 times greater than that of the general male population in that group."

Most physicians, says Dr. Morton, are not familiar with the findings on hypertension incidence in industry. Instead, they relate nitrates with medication for the relief of angina pectoris. Dr. Morton cites proof from many research laboratories which "raise the possibility that therapy with long-acting organic nitrates might hasten the progress of coronary artery disease rather than alleviate it. Clearly, this possibility must be investigated."

Dr. Morton notes a relationship between water nitrate level and the development of hypertension as well as many deaths. "Rural and suburban water sources would seem to be at particular risk of increasing nitrate levels. There is currently no economical method for removing nitrate from drinking water. This may constitute a major ecological problem . . . We need to know if increased hypertension risk is one of the ecological consequences of modern intensive agricultural procedures." He refers to the use of nitrate fertilizers.

If possible, consider drinking bottled water if the water in your area has a high nitrate content. Select organically grown foods, instead of those coming from nitrate-treated fields. Avoid the use of preserved meats or smoked fish. As always, read labels.

CHAPTER SEVEN

HIGH BLOOD PRESSURE AND YOUR KIDNEYS

IT HAS LONG BEEN KNOWN THAT, UNDER CERtain conditions, the kidneys secrete renin, a substance which, when liberated into the bloodstream, causes the production of the hormone *angiotensin*.

Angiotensin narrows the arterioles by constricting their muscular walls. In this way, angiotensin may induce high blood pressure. The kidneys may produce other substances in addition to renin which can cause arteriolar narrowing.

Furthermore, an ailing kidney may fail to perform its normal function of removing from the blood arteriolar-constricting substances produced elsewhere in the body. It appears that hypertension may result from various kinds of kidney malfunction. This begins a vicious cycle, as hypertension injures the kidneys even further and in turn becomes worse. Good kidney health is a bulwark against various forms of hypertension, and basic to body health. Liquids, either water or salt- and sugar-free fruit and vegetable juices, can protect your kidneys and help ward off hypertension. Let us see what the kidneys do to keep you healthy and how you can keep them functioning properly.

THE KIDNEYS—FILTERS OF YOUR BODY SYSTEMS

What are the kidneys? They are bean-shaped organs located in the small of your back (lumbar region) on either side of your spine. Each weighs less than eight ounces and is approximately four inches long, two inches wide and one inch thick.

The kidneys are an extremely complex part of the human machine. They are dedicated to maintaining the chemical balance of the body, the regulating of the volume and the composition of fluids, and the eliminating of harmful substances. They are the super filters of the body.

These amazing filters have specific actions and activities. Each kidney is composed of one to three million tubular structures called nephrons—the basic unit. (A nephron is made up of a tuft of tiny blood vessels, known as glomerulus, and an attached tube or tubule.) As blood enters the kidneys through the renal artery, it is filtered and purified, and returned to the blood system by way of the renal vein. The organs, acting as screens, retain 99 percent of the water and most of the small blood substances and chemical molecules. Waste, as urine, is channeled from the body through the urinary system.

A healthy kidney filters about 200 quarts of blood (three times the body weight in water and salt) every twenty-four hours. It returns some 198 quarts to the bloodstream, producing about seven drops of urine per minute.

The kidneys carry out all of these steps without conscious control. Yet, your kidneys are adaptable. They can adjust to regulate the flow of urine so that during periods of sleep the bladder, which collects the urine, will not fill too rapidly.

As stated above, problems occur when the kidneys do not function properly, especially when they release renin into the bloodstream. This enzyme catalyzes the formation of angiotensin from a plasma protein. That powerful blood-vessel constrictor is the most potent agent known for raising blood pressure. Regular consumption of fresh liquids and juices help to wash out the kidneys and keep them free of toxins and the accumulation of angiotensin.

FLUID FACTS AND NEEDS

Water, that most important liquid, which makes up more than half of your body weight, is constantly being lost and must be replaced. Not all of this water is eliminated as waste. Some is lost in the form of perspiration and unseen and unfelt evaporation through your skin. Some water comes from your lungs. You can see this moisture by breathing on a mirror.

How much liquid do you need? Your need for liquid depends on your size and weight. As a rule, adults should drink between one and a half and two quarts of liquid a day. Children, of course, need proportionately less.

It is important that you drink enough. If you drink too little, the salts and minerals excreted by your kidneys may not be flushed completely from your system. These minerals may cause the formation of kidney stones. Also, many doctors believe that infection-causing bacteria grows more easily if there is an internal water shortage. These conditions predispose to hypertension. Therefore, drinking enough liquid is a natural way to guard against elevated blood pressure.

Balance your liquid intake. It is very important that you balance out your drinking over your waking hours. If you concentrate all your fluids during a two-hour period, your kidneys will excrete the excess quickly and your body will not benefit. Certain types of workers who do not have a handy water supply often think that if they drink a lot of water before work, they will not need any more until the end of the day. Not only is this untrue, it is also dangerous. If you operate on this theory, by the end of the day, your urine will be very concentrated—a favorable situation for kidney malfunction and hypertension.

You don't have to waterlog yourself to replenish your body's water supply. The fruit and vegetable juices you drink supply water to your body as do herbal teas, coffee substitutes, milk and other beverages. In fact, 85 percent of the average person's total fluid intake represents fluids other than water. But if you miss your daily intake of healthful beverages, make up for it with water.

Avoid coffee. Coffee often causes *diuresis*—the medical term for increased urination. If coffee goes "straight through you," then your body is not gaining water from this source. You would do well to use any of the coffee substitutes such as dandelion root, Postum, roasted malt or the popular breakfast cup products available at health food stores.

Avoid alcohol. Alcohol drinks also tend to cause diuresis. The big morning-after thirst is caused by water depletion. Drinks mixed with water or soda do not cause as much depletion as less diluted drinks. But it is best to avoid alcohol in any form.

People who live alone or are retired frequently do not drink enough, simply because a cup of a beverage is not much fun when unaccompanied by conversation. If this describes you, make an extra effort to drink an adequate amount. One way to do this is to follow a drinking schedule until it becomes habit. Drink with meals; take time in mid-morning and mid-afternoon to drink water, juices, coffee substitutes, herbal teas or fermented milk beverages. Have something to sip in the evening while you are reading, listening to the radio or watching television.

Fluid needs vary throughout the day. During exercise or hard work, fluids lost through excessive sweating must be replaced. No one has to tell most people to drink to replace these fluids; when you are tired and hot, you are also thirsty. If you eat a great deal, you need additional fluids to get rid of the extra salt in the food, and to replace fluids that are lost when that food is metabolized.

When you are not eating because of an upset stomach, a diet, or for any other reason, you need to drink more to replace the pint of water that comes from most normal daily food intake.

Increased loss of water from the skin reduces body temperature. Therefore, when you have a fever, you need more fluids.

Salt intake calls for more liquids. If you eat salty foods, you will also need more liquids to excrete the extra salt in the wastes. Usually, salt makes you thirsty, so you automatically drink more. As we have said, it is best to avoid using salt in cooking or seasoning anyway, and to substitute natural, salt-free herbs and spices.

A NUTRITIONAL PROGRAM FOR BETTER KIDNEY HEALTH

The very small kidney tubules are lined with mucous membranes that need to be kept open to perform their self-cleansing action. Vitamin A helps keep these membranes in good working order. Supplements are available; in foods, good vitamin A sources are dairy products, fresh vegetables, liver, lean meats and poultry. Eat them regularly to keep well supplied.

Protein helps replenish lost or damaged kidney cells and tissues, and guards against edema or waterlogging. Daily, eat whole grain foods, lean meats or fish, natural cheeses, eggs, peas, beans, nuts and seeds.

Vitamin C also helps build and maintain healthy kidney tissues. Since this is a water-soluble vitamin, much of it is given off in wastes. Replenish the loss with supplements, fresh fruit juices and fruits.

Vitamin E (alpha tocopherol) is also believed to be helpful in kidney function. The noted physician, Evan Shute, in *The Heart and Vitamin E*, tells us,

"Alpha tocopherol plays a wonderful role in the acute cases [of kidney disease]. It far surpasses any other agent so far used. It may smother the early phase as water smothers a fire. Doses should be large, and other ordinary precautions should be observed about handling the . . . infection. There is real hope, too early yet to state with any assurance, that the rapid resolution of the acute phase of the disease by alpha tocopherol may prevent many of the late or chronic cases from developing, and thus may prevent some hypertensions in later life." Vitamin E is available in capsule form. It is also found in whole grain foods, especially wheat germ.

Nutritionist Adelle Davis, in *Let's Get Well*, draws from medical sources for a program to nourish the kidneys (and body) and promote resistance to hypertension. Here is the program:

Protein. From 150 to 200 grams of protein daily.

Sodium restriction. Select low-sodium milk and cheeses. Torula yeast is especially low in sodium. Available low-sodium products are wheat germ, soybeans, soy flour, nuts and salt-free nut butters.

(Oils should be used for cooking and in salads, instead of hydrogenated or hard fats.)

Supplements. If meat is permitted, fresh and/or desiccated liver should be taken several times daily, particularly if anemia is present.

Adelle Davis also suggests taking daily:

1. From 3 to 6 tablespoons of lecithin and 1000 milligrams of choline, usually as 250 milligrams at each meal and before bed
2. 30 milligrams or more of vitamin B_6
3. 25,000 units of natural vitamin A
4. From 300 to 600 units of vitamin E
5. 250 milligrams of calcium four to six times a day if milk is not included in the diet
6. Include some magnesium and 10 milligrams of vitamin B_2

Mrs. Davis writes: "The success of a nutrition program depends largely on how promptly dietary improvement is initiated. If an adequate diet is given from the moment the diagnosis is made, the usual attitude that kidney diseases are 'not amenable to cure' appears to be unjustified. If given a chance, our bodies have an amazing ability to heal themselves."

A variety of kidney-soothing beverages. To protect yourself from hypertension, drink a variety of fresh fruit and vegetable juices. You may prefer to squeeze your own from seasonal plants rather than use bottled juices. If so, you can obtain an electric juice extractor for convenient preparation.

You may also enjoy salt-free, sugar-free and caffeine-free beverages in bottles and cans, available at health stores. These include:

Tiger's Milk, either plain or flavored. Carob beverages. Grapefruit, apple, grape, blackberry, tomato, orange, pineapple, prune, celery, beet, carrot, sauerkraut, apricot, black cherry, cabbage, cherry, raspberry, boysenberry, papaya, fig juice, to name just a few.

Also available are soy milk products, milk substitutes, non-fat dry milk products, goat's milk, cereal beverages, Swiss-style coffee substitutes, dandelion root, breakfast cup beverages.

Round out your thirst quenching with an assortment of herb teas. The variety is almost infinite: peppermint, fenugreek, alfalfa, rose hip, fennel, chamomile, comfrey, flaxseed, golden seal, hyssop, marjoram, papaya, raspberry, red clover, sarsaparilla, senna leaves, slippery elm bark, spearmint, watercress, yarrow.

These and many more healthful beverages are available to boost your basic health, and help free your body from excessive sugar, salt, caffeine and other destructive substances.

A basic function of the kidneys is to regulate the

acidity and alkalinity of body fluids. They do this by retaining or releasing substances according to conditions required to establish the optimum level.

This balance of body fluids prevents the release of excess renin, and is an effective way to avoid the development of hypertension.

CHAPTER EIGHT

NATURAL WAYS TO CONTROL STRESS

NOISE POLLUTION CAN CREATE A STRESS-TEN-sion situation that elevates your blood pressure. *Noise can make you sick!* According to Dr. Leo L. Beranek, a leading accoustical authority, "The noises of our daily life have been blamed variously for the high divorce rate, social conflict, indigestion and other organic disabilities, high blood pressure, heart failure and even insanity. Most of these ills can be attributed just as easily to other causes, but one cannot rule out the possibility that some people are particularly sensitive to noise just as others are allergic to nuts, eggs or dust!"

The *Medical World News* tells us, "To the clinician, noise pollution is as much a threat to certain persons as air pollution is to asthmatics or persons with emphysema. Studies have shown that prolonged exposure to noise or sudden sharp noise produces involuntary responses by the vascular, digestive and nervous systems. The danger to hearing is obvious, but the more subtle physiological and emotional responses to noise place the physician in the position of having to advise the person to remove himself to a quieter environment."

Excessive noise can cause blood pressure to shoot up to an unhealthy high. Samuel Rosen, M.D., of New York's Mt. Sinai Hospital and a specialist in problems of noise pollution, paints this unhealthy picture:

"Epinephrine (adrenalin; the emergency hormone produced by one part of the adrenal glands) is shot into the blood during stress and anxiety. The heart beats rapidly, the blood vessels constrict, the pupils dilate, the head turns, the skin pales and the stomach, esophagus and intestines are seized by spasms. When the noise is prolonged there are heart flutters that eventually subside when the noise diminishes.

"The body's reactions to sudden sounds that leap out in sharp contrast to background noise can be measured. More difficult to ascertain is the effect of noise on the psyche. Does it produce mental and emotional problems in people exposed to noise pollution?"

Scientists feel that noise can cause the reactions that cause hypertension.

The *Medical World News* tells us, "Some psychiatrists and psychologists believe that in the unusually high noise levels—traffic, sirens, police whistles, noisy children, blaring television sets and transistor radios—in the slums, just one extra startle sound may often trigger violence. Even in quiet suburbia, the man who comes home after a tense, stressful day in noisy environment may say nothing when he discovers the kids camped in front of an inordinately loud television set. He may not even react consciously to his daughter's phonograph. Then, a child will accidentally drop a toy, or the telephone will ring, or his wife will yell suddenly at a child—and he flares up wrathfully."

Noise causes a "fear reaction" in your body. Sound is instantly transmitted from your ears to your brain and then to your nerves, glands and body organs. Any loud or unexpected sounds put your body on alert. Noise means trouble to your body and it instantly readies itself for defense. You react to sudden noises in the same way you react to being frightened.

Constant response to these alerts or false alarms raises blood pressure. Stress and nervousness result. Over a period of years, these reactions can lead to heart disease, high blood pressure, chronic headaches and ulcers.

Steady noise causes hypertension. Steady levels of noise also have harmful effects. While you may not have the same fear reaction as with sudden noise, your nerves are still affected. You develop hypertension, become irritable and may eventually suffer from emotional as well as physical stress.

Noise causes tension while you sleep. Sounds not loud enough to awaken you with a start can still interrupt dreams and cause you to wake up feeling exhausted. Prolonged sleep loss can eventually contribute to hypertension.

Most noise pollution in larger cities comes from cars, trucks, motorcycles, buses, sirens, horn honking, power machines, drills, aircraft and subways. Items in the home also contribute to noise pollution: loud radios and stereos, appliances, alarm clocks and typewriters. Barking dogs, hammering and screaming are nuisance noises that contribute to hypertension.

The following chart shows some noise levels you are exposed to as well as the typical response to each level. "dBA" stands for "decibel" on the A scale, the unit used for measuring sound. Noise doubles approximately every 10 dBA; 90 dBA is therefore twice as loud as 80 dBA.

HOW TO HELP CONTROL NOISE POLLUTION

Immediate steps to take include:

Put carpets on the upper floors of your house to deaden the noise of footsteps.

Use heavy drapes in front of noisy windows or walls to absorb noise from outside and reduce the reverberations of sounds within the room.

Use upholstered furniture and accoustical ceilings to minimize noise.

Seal windows to keep down outside noise.

Silence noisy plumbing by inserting neoprene or cork where pipes connect with other solid structures.

Replace loose or worn faucet washers to eliminate whistling or chattering noises.

Lower the setting on the heater thermostat to eliminate noises caused by very hot water.

Kitchen noises are hazardous; hypertension can be eased by creating a peaceful home. Dr. Lee E. Farr of the California Department of Health explains, "The ventilating fan over the stove, the dishwasher, the garbage disposal unit, the blender, all make significant contributions to sound, which steel cabinets and hard surfaces reflect, augment and cause to reverberate.

"A tired, taut person will certainly not leave a kitchen pleasantly relaxed; nor do the roars, squeaks,

EFFECTS OF EVERYDAY SOUNDS ON TENSION

SOURCE	NOISE LEVEL dBA		EFFECT ON SPEECH	HEARING IMPAIRMENT
POWER DRILL	140			Acute pain
	130			
JET TAKE-OFF (200 feet)	120			
AUTO HORN (3 feet)	110	Hearing damage at ½ hr. per day		
TYPICAL SUBWAY NOISE	100	Hearing damage at 2 hrs. per day	Shouting in ear	Discomfort
FOOD BLENDER HEAVY TRUCK (25 feet)	90	Hearing damage at 8 hours per day	Shouting at 2 feet	Very annoying
HEAVY TRAFFIC (RUSH HOUR)	85		Very loud conversation at 2 feet	
ALARM CLOCK (3 feet)	80			
VACUUM CLEANER (10 feet)	70	Telephone use difficult Noisy	Loud conversation 2 feet	Annoyance Threshold
AVERAGE HOME	50	Quiet	Normal conversation 12 feet	Sleep interference
WHISPER	30	Very quiet		
BREATHING	10	Threshold of hearing		
	0			

Source: New York City Department of Health

whirrs and whines issuing from it lead to quiet contemplation of pleasant meals by those who are waiting. Home sounds can threaten the health and well-being of one's emotional state."

NUTRITION CAN EASE STRESS AND HYPERTENSION

An effective nutritional program can strengthen the body to help meet the onslaught of daily stress and tension. Nutrition acts as a stress-shield to insulate the nervous system and keep blood pressure under control.

The B-complex vitamins. Dr. Roger J. Williams, author of *Nutrition in a Nutshell,* singles out thiamine (B_1), niacin, B_{12} and pantothenic acid as the specifics of the B-complex family for this purpose. Without these, the nerve cells develop severe abnormalities in function. "This is another example in which failure of cells to get what they need in one area can cause nerve damage elsewhere in the body," says Dr. Williams.

Good sources of the B-complex group include whole grain, non-processed wheat products, meat, eggs, dried beans and peas, natural and organic nut butters of all types and whole-grain cereals.

Calcium. This valuable mineral helps transmit impulses along nerves. According to Drs. Best and Taylor, in the *Physiological Basis of Medical Practice,* a calcium deficiency leads to nervous disorders. Take calcium tablets, or select such natural food sources as: milk, cheese (there is less calcium in cottage cheese) turnip and mustard greens, collards, kale, broccoli.

Adelle Davis in *Let's Eat Right To Keep Fit,* offers this nerve-soothing calcium program:

"If you drink daily one quart of skim milk fortified with powdered milk, and if you take calcium tablets before meals, the nervousness, insomnia and leg cramps resulting from calcium deficiency will probably soon disappear. When sleeplessness and nocturnal leg cramps are problems, it is often wise to take calcium tablets just before retiring; keep the tablets by your bedside and take more during the night if wakeful or if leg cramps recur."

Protein-vitamin. "There is no doubt protein is important, but protein is not the only nutrient affecting emotional health, nor is it the only one of which malnourished people fail to get enough." So spoke A. A. Pokrovsky, M.D., at the International Conference on Malnutrition, Learning and Behavior at the Massachusetts Institute of Technology. "Even though not every nutrient is directly involved in the development of the nervous system, malnutrition of any type will cause malfunctioning of the metabolism and that will affect the health and abilities of the brain."

Dr. Pokrovsky suggests niacin and protein supplements to be given for disorders arising from hypertension.

You can eat your way to better emotional health. Wholesome, natural foods can do much to help soothe your nervous system and calm tense emotions. To repeat: enjoy fresh fruits and vegetables, fresh juices, organic meats, fish, eggs, nuts and seeds. Take supplements—brewer's yeast, desiccated liver, kelp, and the many vitamin-mineral-protein supplements to be used in conjunction with your doctor's approval. Select unadulterated, unprocessed, unsalted foods. Finally, avoid harmful stimulants—caffeine, tobacco and alcohol.

EIGHT WAYS TO HELP LOWER HIGH BLOOD PRESSURE

There are no easy ways to control everyday strain and stress. Experience is the best teacher. Learn how to cope, how to relieve daily tension with some of these suggestions:

1. *Balance work with play.* If you have trouble relaxing long enough to enjoy life, then schedule time for recreation. For many people, an interesting hobby can be relaxing as well as constructive. On the other hand, work can often be a kind of healing for emotional situations hard to bear. Keeping busy often relieves tension and, therefore, high blood pressure.

2. *Loaf . . . it's good for you.* Very active people who feel guilty about just sitting and doing plain nothing occasionally should give themselves a chance to learn and enjoy the art of loafing. While too much inactivity breeds boredom and may even cause stress, a little bit of doing nothing may help you back to work with renewed enthusiasm. By slowing down a bit, you may be able to enjoy more fully the better things of life.

3. *Get enough sleep and rest.* Continued lack of sleep causes hypertension. No one can enjoy good health for long without enough sleep and rest. Most people need seven or eight hours of sleep a night. The best test of your sleeping needs is how you feel. If you awake refreshed and energetic, you are getting adequate rest. But if you feel tired and often out of sorts, the solution may well be as simple as going to bed earlier and being as regular as possible in your sleep habits. Scientific studies show that cumulative sleep loss contributes to high blood pressure. Of

course, worry and tension can interfere with a good night's sleep. Although most people have an occasional restless night, chronic inability to sleep should be discussed with a physician and nutritional therapy considered.

4. *Work off tensions.* When you are upset or angry, you can often work off your feelings with physical exercise. Pitching into some activity, like working in the garden, taking a long walk or playing a game of tennis or some other sport not only relieves anger but makes it easier to face and handle irritating problems more calmly. Regular exercise is also a great way to keep yourself in good physical condition.

5. *Talk it out.* It helps to get worry off your chest by talking to a sympathetic listener. When what appears to be a serious problem gets you down, it is sensible to discuss it with your doctor, clergyman, a friend or an understanding member of your family. Often another person can help you see your problem in a new light. This may be the first step toward a constructive solution.

6. *Learn to accept.* That is: accept what you cannot change. Many people become upset about circumstances beyond control. Sometimes, they even try to make people over to fit their own demands and then feel frustrated or let down on discovering that this is not possible. Look for the best in others. Realize that no one is perfect—not even yourself!

7. *Get away from it all.* When you feel that you are going around in circles with a problem or a worry, try to divert yourself. As simple a thing as going to the movies, reading a story or visiting a friend can help you out of a rut. There is no

harm in running away from a hypertensive situation long enough to catch your breath and regain the composure to come back and face the problem. When possible and practical, a change of scene can give a new perspective. There are times when we all need to escape—even for just a brief letup from routine. Certainly everyone should have a few hours to call his own, away from immediate cares and worries. For many of us, this means a few moments just to be alone.

8. *Avoid disagreeable situations.* Steer clear of irritating situations as much as you can. Avoid meaningless conflicts. Avoid stress-tensions. Whenever possible, try to protect yourself against the onslaught of hypertensive irritants. You'll feel better!

CHAPTER NINE

FOODS THAT HELP CONTROL HYPERTENSION

SOME FOODS REALLY DO SOOTHE BODY AND mind and help diminish those physiological reactions that raise blood pressure. When they are included in the diet they provide natural, easy ways to help control hypertension. Here are a few of these valuable foods:

GARLIC—FOLKLORE HYPERTENSION HEALER

In the European medical journal, *Praxis*, a physician-member of the faculty of medicine at the University of Geneva praises the value of garlic as a help for hypertension. G. Piotrowski, M.D. writes of his experiences with the use of garlic on "about a hundred patients."

Dr. Piotrowski contends that garlic lowers blood pressure by dilating the blood vessels. He further reports that garlic helps cleanse the intestines of waste products; and while he says this does not have a direct influence on lowering pressure, it improves the general health of the body and this in turn helps control blood pressure. Since hypertension has many causes, toxemia could very well be one of the contributing factors.

Two New York doctors use garlic as a natural healer. In the *New York Physician,* Drs. David Stein and Edward H. Kotin explain that garlic is a prime source of vitamins A, B and C. Garlic also has good mineral content, including manganese, copper, zinc, sulfur, iron, calcium and natural chlorine. These doctors feel that garlic is therapeutically useful as a cleanser.

Drs. Klein and Kotin say that garlic has other healing properties. It helps stimulate the gastric juices. It is a fine carminative, which means that it eases digestive unrest and creates a better emotional and physical mood. It is believed helpful in respiratory infections, especially those signified by a dry hacking cough. It is said to have value as a nerve tonic and because it can soothe neurasthenia and nerve insufficiency, it may therefore help the control of hypertension.

The doctors cite a number of cases treated with garlic with good results. Relief was often noted within a week, always within a month, on garlic therapy. "In conclusion," say the physicians, "we feel that garlic is an excellent medicament for employment in a diversity of conditions. We believe that the vitamin and mineral factors do much to cause this to be a 'drug' of noteworthy usage."

Garlic should be used regularly in raw salads. Garlic perles or tablets are also available, alone or with parsley (a helpful nutritional companion), and should be considered as a simple source of improved well-being.

DAIRY PRODUCTS ARE BENEFICIAL

The calcium and phosphorus in dairy products can be very soothing to the nervous system. The hypertensive should consider the use of milk, cheese, yogurt, kefir and other such healthful foods. If you are on a doctor-supervised low-sodium, low-fat program, ask about the feasibility of using salt-free dairy products, as well as salt-free milk products. These are currently available in many health stores and other outlets.

A glass of skim milk with a fresh fruit salad will give your body a supply of needed minerals that act in a soothing capacity and help control the circumstances contributing to an elevated blood pressure. Yogurt made from skim milk, kefir milk or low-fat cheeses also provide these valuable minerals. As a means of hypertension control and general good health, some dairy products should be part of your daily diet.

WHOLE GRAINS OFFER NATURAL VITALITY

Many a hypertensive is nervous or jumpy and this is often misinterpreted for energy. It may be a throbbing, persistent, blood-pounding urgency that can lead to serious complications if not controlled.

Whole grains assist the body's energy capacity, supplying natural rather than nervous energy. They should, of course, be prepared without salt.

Oats, millet, bran and wheat germ alone or combined at breakfast, a whole-grain bread at lunch, brown rice, unpearled barley or bulgur wheat at dinner, are all most helpful in providing the very best carbohydrates for the body to use. These *natural* carbohydrates are not to be confused with the useless sugar and refined flour that cause erratic blood sugar and internal upheaval. Schedule these wholesome foods daily in the menu.

ALMONDS

Almonds are one of the best of all nuts and a prime source of protein. They often substitute for meat; they help give the body needed amino acids and are free of the saturated fats in meat.

Go on a meatless day—or even two-day—schedule. Try a main course of a large raw vegetable salad with almonds; it will give you much-needed nutrition and help reduce hypertension.

APPLES AND APPLE JUICE

The malic acid content in apples appears to work as a fine relaxant. Try to enjoy apples and apple juice regularly. You may make your own apple juice with an electric extractor or drink bottled or canned apple juice. You can also mix apple with other fruit juices for nutritional balance. Pure juices are available at health stores.

BEANS AND LEGUMES

Beans and legumes are very high in protein, vitamin and mineral content. They may be eaten as vegetables, steamed with a bit of oil. They may also be sprouted for a concentrated form of vital nutrients. Seed sprouters are available at health stores as are the seeds and beans for sprouting. These excellent sources of natural carbohydrates provide energy and reduce the need for artificial stimulants.

They also help promote body balance and soothe the nervous system. They are delicious *without* salt.

BERRIES

Seasonal berries and their juices are extremely valuable sources of the vitamins and minerals which indirectly temper hypertension. They are available in bottled form in health stores if you can't get them fresh. Add raw berries to fruit salads; drink their juices frequently.

CABBAGE

An important source of vitamins and minerals, cabbage also contains a yet-to-be-identified factor in its juices that seems to soothe nervous stomachs and ulcerous conditions. It is believed to improve relaxation and tranquility, both important in hypertensive problems.

Eat lightly steamed cabbage regularly as your vegetable. (It is very good with yogurt as a sauce.) Prepare cabbage juice from the raw vegetable; drink it as a cocktail. Again, *no* salt in cooking, eating raw or drinking the juice.

PINEAPPLE

A delightful fruit that is an excellent source of vitamins, minerals and, particularly, raw enzymes. These nutrients in the fruit and juice provide better digestive metabolism and overall body assimilation. Hypertension is eased when the digestive mechanisms are in good working condition. If internal clogging is relieved, the whole body feels better.

Pineapple in fruit salad, or as dessert with sun-dried fruits and seeds and nuts is always refreshing; and its juice, especially when taken during respiratory infections, is not only nourishing and relaxing, but therapeutic.

SEAFOOD

Fresh fish is a prime source of the unsaturated fatty acids that help lower blood cholesterol and give protection against high blood pressure. Many physicians recommend fish (excluding shellfish) as a substitute for meat at least three times a week. Steam it, bake it, broil it, serve it with a raw vegetable salad and fresh fruit dessert and you have one of the healthiest, most delicious meals possible.

GENERAL RULES:

Chemical additives in foods tend to elevate the blood pressure. Foods should be as natural and organic as possible, and this means raw whenever it is feasible. If necessary to cook, do so without additives or harsh, volatile seasonings. Use herbs and other natural seasonings. If you bear in mind the dictum that Nature can keep you cool, calm and collected, you can eat your way to better moods and controlled hypertension.

CHAPTER TEN

REDUCE—AND LOWER
YOUR BLOOD PRESSURE

OVERWEIGHT IS USUALLY ACCOMPANIED BY an increase in blood pressure because of the added circulatory workload that obesity imposes on the heart.

Blood volume increases with body weight. Moreover, adipose tissue, like organ and muscle tissues, must be supplied with blood. It has been estimated that each extra pound of fat requires about a mile of capillaries to nourish it. Thus, in obese persons, the heart is forced to pump more blood through a more extensive system of blood vessels.

The elevated blood pressure resulting from obesity appears to be chiefly responsible for the increased susceptibility of overweight people to coronary heart disease and stroke, findings from the Heart Institute's Framingham Study indicate.

This long-term study of factors affecting the development of coronary heart disease and cerebrovascular disease in a population of 5,127 Americàn adults reveals that risk of angina pectoris and sudden death increases with the degree of overweight.

Obesity problem. Among those who were more than 20 percent overweight, the risk was approximately three times that of non-obese or underweight individuals. Obesity also appears to increase risk of stroke, though to a much lesser degree.

The overweight person with hypertension should be placed on a reducing diet by his physician. It is a recognized fact that weight reduction lowers blood pressure.

SO YOU WANT TO LOSE WEIGHT? HERE'S HOW . . .

Diets by the hundreds . . . recipes by the thousands . . . mountains of books and pamphlets and folders and charts—all advising you how to slim down to glamorous proportions. Yet the fact remains that dieting to lose weight is difficult for most of us.

What works? Will power helps, of course. And so does the advice of nutritionists and other scientists who have devoted careful study to weight control. If you want to lose and lose successfully, start with the essentials. Read on:

Cut down, not out. Eat fewer calories than your body requires to maintain your weight and you will inevitably lose. This doesn't mean singling out one or two foods with high-calorie reputations and dropping them from your life. It does mean eating less of everything, without skipping the daily food essentials.

Forget about crash diets. They just don't work in the long run. The pounds you lose are soon regained and sometimes even increased—when you return to normal eating habits. Furthermore, your health (to say nothing of your looks and your disposition) can be impaired by repeated diet binges.

Make haste slowly. The only safe sure way to lose is to take off the ounces that add up to pounds. Weight lost slowly usually stays lost, for you gradually (almost unconsciously) change your eating habits. Chances are that you'll never go back to eating as much as before. In fact, you may even wonder how you ever ate that much in the first place.

ARE YOU OVERWEIGHT?

Since people come in a variety of sizes and shapes, large-boned or small-boned, firm muscled or flaccid, short and stocky or tall and lanky, with many variations in between, no one weight is exactly right for everyone of the same height and sex.

The weight that is best for you depends upon your individual frame size and muscular development. It is the weight at which you look and feel your best. Some people look and feel better when they weigh somewhat more than their statistically-desirable weight, if the extra weight is largely firm muscle, not fat.

One way to determine whether too much of your weight is just fat is by pinching the back of your upper arm. If you can pinch a thickness of one inch or more, chances are you are carrying excess fat—and excess weight. (This test is most meaningful for persons under fifty years of age.) If you are 20 percent above your desirable weight, your physician probably will recommend that you start losing weight.

The following table is a general guide to the best (that is, healthy) weights for men and women at age twenty-five and over:

MEN

HEIGHT (with shoes on) 1-inch heels		SMALL FRAME	MEDIUM FRAME	LARGE FRAME
Feet	Inches			
5	2	112–120	118–129	126–141
5	3	115–123	121–133	129–144
5	4	118–126	124–136	132–148
5	5	121–129	127–139	135–152
5	6	124–133	130–143	138–156
5	7	128–137	134–147	142–161
5	8	132–141	138–152	147–166
5	9	136–145	142–156	151–170
5	10	140–150	146–160	155–174
5	11	144–154	150–165	159–179
6	0	148–158	154–170	164–184
6	1	152–162	158–175	168–189
6	2	156–167	162–180	173–194
6	3	160–171	167–185	178–199
6	4	164–175	172–190	182–204

HOW MANY CALORIES DO YOU NEED?

The daily calorie needs shown in the tables in this chapter are only for your guidance. The calorie needs of no two people are alike. In addition to height and age, your daily calorie requirement depends upon body frame, present weight, desired weight, occupational activities and other daily activities at home and at play.

The calorie needs in these tables are averages based on studies of women and men of normal weight engaged in moderate activity. Housewives,

WOMEN

HEIGHT (with shoes on) 2-inch heels		SMALL FRAME	MEDIUM FRAME	LARGE FRAME
Feet	Inches			
4	10	92– 98	96–107	104–119
4	11	94–101	98–110	106–122
5	0	96–104	101–113	109–125
5	1	99–107	104–116	112–128
5	2	102–110	107–119	115–131
5	3	105–113	110–122	118–134
5	4	108–116	113–126	121–138
5	5	111–119	116–130	125–142
5	6	114–123	120–135	129–146
5	7	118–127	124–139	133–150
5	8	122–131	128–143	137–154
5	9	126–135	132–147	141–158
5	10	130–140	136–151	145–163
5	11	134–144	140–155	149–168
6	0	138–148	144–159	153–173

For girls between 18 and 25, subtract 1 pound for each year under 25.

Weight in Pounds According to Frame (In Indoor Clothing)

Source: Metropolitan Life Insurance Company

clerical workers and workers in light industry are included.

If you are in an occupation that requires heavy physical activity, you may be able to use anywhere from 10 percent to 20 percent more calories than indicated here, without gaining weight. If you are retired or homebound and not too active, your calorie needs could be 10 percent less than indicated.

The tables also take into consideration the fact that younger people are more active generally. For example, 60 percent of the calorie requirements of those between fifteen and nineteen years of age are

DAILY CALORIE NEEDS FOR MEN OF NORMAL WEIGHT*

Height	Age 15–19	Age 20–29	Age 30–39	Age 40–49	Age 50–59	Age 60–69	Age 70–79
5ft. 0	2,620	2,250	2,100	2,020	1,980	1,710	1,570
5ft. 1in.	2,690	2,310	2,160	2,070	2,020	1,750	1,610
5ft. 2in.	2,750	2,390	2,220	2,110	2,070	1,790	1,650
5ft. 3in.	2,820	2,450	2,280	2,160	2,110	1,830	1,690
5ft. 4in.	2,880	2,500	2,340	2,200	2,160	1,880	1,740
5ft. 5in.	2,940	2,560	2,400	2,260	2,200	1,920	1,780
5ft. 6in.	3,000	2,620	2,460	2,320	2,250	1,950	1,810
5ft. 7in.	3,070	2,680	2,520	2,380	2,310	2,000	1,850
5ft. 8in.	3,140	2,740	2,580	2,440	2,370	2,060	1,900
5ft. 9in.	3,200	2,800	2,640	2,500	2,430	2,100	1,930
5ft. 10in.	3,280	2,880	2,710	2,560	2,490	2,160	1,990
5ft. 11in.	3,360	2,950	2,790	2,620	2,550	2,210	2,040
6ft. 0	3,440	3,030	2,860	2,680	2,610	2,250	2,070
6ft. 1in.	3,520	3,130	2,940	2,740	2,670	2,310	2,130
6ft. 2in.	3,600	3,180	3,010	2,800	2,730	2,370	2,180
6ft. 3in.	3,680	3,250	3,090	2,860	2,790	2,410	2,220

allocated for physical activity, and only 40 percent for those past sixty.

These tables were developed by Norman Jolliffe, M.D., who gained an international reputation as Director of the Bureau of Nutrition, New York City Department of Health.

How calories can be lost. Think of your body as a bank in which you can deposit or withdraw calories. You deposit calories by eating. You withdraw them in the form of energy. When your account is balanced, so is your weight. In other words, your weight is maintained.

Your calorie/energy account is a personal thing. The calories you need are directly related to the kind

DAILY CALORIE NEEDS FOR WOMEN OF NORMAL WEIGHT*

Height	Age 15–19	Age 20–29	Age 30–39	Age 40–49	Age 50–59	Age 60–69	Age 70–79
4ft. 9in.	2,080	1,890	1,810	1,760	1,710	1,480	1,370
4ft. 10in.	2,110	1,920	1,840	1,790	1,740	1,510	1,400
4ft. 11in.	2,140	1,950	1,870	1,820	1,770	1,530	1,430
5ft. 0	2,190	1,980	1,900	1,850	1,800	1,550	1,450
5ft. 1in.	2,240	2,020	1,940	1,890	1,850	1,590	1,480
5ft. 2in.	2,290	2,060	1,980	1,950	1,900	1,640	1,510
5ft. 3in.	2,350	2,100	2,030	2,000	1,950	1,690	1,550
5ft. 4in.	2,400	2,150	2,080	2,040	2,000	1,740	1,590
5ft. 5in.	2,460	2,200	2,140	2,080	2,050	1,780	1,640
5ft. 6in.	2,520	2,250	2,190	2,120	2,100	1,820	1,690
5ft. 7in.	2,570	2,300	2,240	2,160	2,150	1,860	1,730
5ft. 8in.	2,620	2,350	2,290	2,220	2,200	1,910	1,770
5ft. 9in.	2,680	2,400	2,340	2,260	2,250	1,950	1,800
5ft. 10in.	2,740	2,450	2,400	2,310	2,300	1,990	1,830
5ft. 11in.	2,800	2,500	2,450	2,360	2,350	2,040	1,880
6ft. 0	2,860	2,550	2,500	2,410	2,400	2,090	1,930

*This intake will generally maintain normal weight at present level.

Source: U.S. Public Health Service

of person you are and the kind of physical activities in which you are involved.

The best way to keep your calorie/energy account balanced is to make certain that the number of calories you take into your body is about equal to the number of calories you use up in your daily activities. When the calories you use up in the form of energy are higher in amount than the calories that you eat, the difference is known as the calorie deficit. The larger your deficit, the greater your weight loss. A deficit of 3500 calories means the loss of one pound of weight.

Doctors recommend that you lose weight slowly, at the rate of no more than two pounds per week. By eating less you force your body to consume the extra calories it has stored in the form of fat, thus burning away those extra pounds.

To maintain your weight, you need 15 calories for every pound. If you weigh 150 pounds, you need 2250 calories a day just to keep your weight where it is. But if you want to reduce, you must cut out 3500 calories for every pound you want to lose. Therefore, to lose two pounds a week, you must cut out 7000 calories a week or 1000 calories a day. So if you weigh 150 pounds and want to weigh 140, in order to lose two pounds a week you must reduce your daily calorie intake from 2250 to 1250 for five weeks.

CALORIE TABLES

1 cup equals 8 fluid ounces. 3 teaspoons (tsp.) equal 1 tablespoon (tbs.). 4 tablespoons (tbs.) equal ¼ cup.

Food and Measures	Approximate Calories
A	
Almonds....12–15	100
Apple butter....1 tbs.	40
Apples	
baked....1 lg. and 2 tbs. sugar	200
fresh....1 large	100
Applesauce, sweetened ½ cup.	100
Apricots	
canned in syrup....3 lg. halves and 2 tbs. juice	100
dried..10 sm. halves	100

Food and Measures	Approximate Calories
Asparagus	
fresh or canned....5 stalks 5 ins. long	15
Avocado....½ pear 3½ x 3¼ ins.	185
B	
Bacon....2–3 long slices, cooked	100
Bacon fat....1 tbs.	100
Banana....1 med., 6 ins. long	90
Beans	
canned with pork ½ cup	175

Food and Measures	Approximate Calories
dried..½ cup, cooked	135
lima, fresh or canned ½ cup	100
snap, fresh or canned ½ cup	25
Beef (cooked)	
corned....1 slice 4 by 1½ by 1 ins.	100
dried....2 ozs.	100
hamburger....1 patty (3 ozs.)	300
round, lean....1 med. slice (2 ozs.)	125
sirloin, lean....1 av. slice (3 ozs.)	250
tongue....2 ozs.	125
Beet greens....½ cup, cooked	30
Beets, fresh or canned 2 beets 2 ins. in diam.	50
Biscuit, baking powder 2 ins. in diam.	100
Blackberries, fresh 1 cup	100
Blueberries, fresh 1 cup	90
Bologna....1 slice 2 ins. by ½ in. thick	100
Breads	
Boston brown....1 slice 3 ins. in diam. ¾ in. thick	90
corn (1-egg) 1 2-in. square	120
cracked wheat 1 slice, av.	80
dark rye....1 slice ½ in. thick	70
light rye....1 slice ½ in. thick	75

Food and Measures	Approximate Calories
white, enriched 1 slice, av.	75
white, enriched 1 slice, thin	55
whole wheat, 60% 1 slice, av.	70
whole wheat, 100% 1 slice, av.	75
Broccoli....3 stalks 5½ ins. long	100
Brownies....1 piece 2 by 2 by ¾ ins.	140
Brussels sprouts 6 sprouts 1½ ins. in diam.	50
Butter....1 tbs.	95

C

Food and Measures	Approximate Calories
Cabbage, cooked.... ½ cup	40
raw....1 cup	25
Cake	
angel....1/10 of a lg. cake	155
chocolate or vanilla, no icing....1 piece 2 by 2 by 2 ins.	200
chocolate or vanilla, with icing....1 piece 2 by 1½ by 2 ins.	200
cupcake with chocolate icing....1 medium	250
Cantaloupe....½ of a 5½-in. melon	50
Carrots....1 carrot 4 ins. long	25
Cashew nuts....4-5	100
Cauliflower....¼ of a hd. 4½ ins. in diam.	25

Food and Measures	Approximate Calories
Caviar....1 tbs.	25
Celery....2 stalks	15
Cheese	
American cheddar	
1 cube 1⅛ ins. square	
or 3 tbs. grated	110
cottage....5 tbs.	100
cream....2 tbs.	100
Cherries, sweet....15 lg.	75
Chicken	
broiled....½ med.	
broiler	270
roast....1 slice	
4 by 2½ by ¼ ins.	100
Chinese cabbage	
1 cup raw	20
Chocolate	
milk, sweetened....	
1 oz.	140
fudge....1 piece 1 in. sq.	
by ¾ in. thick	100
malted milk....fountain	
size	460
mints....1 mint	
1½ ins. in diam.	100
milk with almonds,	
sweetened....1 oz.	150
syrup....¼ cup	200
unsweetened	
1 square	160
Cider, sweet....1 cup	100
Clams....6 round	100
Cocoa, half milk, half	
water....1 cup	150
Coconut....½ cup, fresh	175
Cod-liver oil....1 tbs.	100
Cod steak....1 piece	
3½ by 2 by 1 in.	100
Cola soft drinks	
6-oz. bottle	75

Food and Measures	Approximate Calories
Collards....½ cup,	
cooked	50
Cooking fats, vegetable	
1 tbs.	100
Corn....½ cup	70
Corn syrup....1 tbs.	75
Corn flakes....1 cup	80
Corn meal....1 tbs.,	
uncooked	35
Cornstarch pudding	
½ cup	200
Crackers	
graham....1 square	35
peanut butter-cheese	
sandwich....1 cracker	45
round snack-type	
1 cracker 2 in.	
in diam.	15
rye wafers....1 wafer	25
saltines....1 cracker	
2 ins. sq.	15
Cranberry sauce....	
¼ cup	100
Cream	
light....2 tbs.	65
heavy....2 tbs.	120
whipped....3 tbs.	100
Cream-puff shells....	
1 shell	85
Cucumber....	
½ medium	10
Custard, boiled or baked	
½ cup	130

D

Dates....4	100

E

Egg....1 medium size	75

Food and Measures	Approximate Calories
Eggplant....*3 slices 4 ins. in diam. ½ in. thick, raw*	50
Endive....*average serving*	10
Escarole....*average serving*	10

F

Figs, dried....*3 small*	100
Flour, white or whole grain *1 tbs., unsifted*	35
Frankfurter.... *1 sausage*	125

G

Gelatin, fruit flavored, dry *3 oz. pkg.*	330
ready to serve....*½ cup*	85
Ginger ale....*1 cup*	85
Gingerbread, hot water *2 by 2 by 2 ins.*	200
Grapefruit....*½ medium*	50
Grapefruit juice, unsweetened....*1 cup*	100
Grape juice....*½ cup*	80
Grape nuts....*¼ cup*	100
Grapes American or Tokay *1 bunch—22, av.*	75
seedless....*1 bunch— 30, av.*	75
Griddle cakes *1 cake 4 ins. in diam.*	75

H

Halibut....*1 piece 3 by 1⅜ by 1 ins.*	100

Food and Measures	Approximate Calories
Ham, lean....*1 slice 4¼ by 4 by ½ ins.*	265
Hard sauce....*1 tbs.*	100
Hickory nuts....*12–15*	100
Hominy grits *¾ cup, cooked*	100
Honey....*1 tbs.*	100

I

Ice cream....*½ cup*	200
Ice cream soda *fountain size*	325

J

Jellies and jams *1 rounded tbs.*	100

K

Kale....*½ cup, cooked*	50

L

Lamb, roast....*1 slice 3½ by 4½ by ⅛ ins.*	100
Lard....*1 tbs.*	100
Lemon juice....*1 tbs.*	5
Lettuce....*2 lg. leaves*	5
Liver....*1 slice 3 by 3 by ½ ins.*	100
Liverwurst....*2 ozs.*	130
Lobster meat....*1 cup*	150

M

Macaroni....*¾ cup, cooked*	100
Maple syrup....*1 tbs.*	70
Margarine....*1 tbs.*	100
Marshmallows....*1*	20
Milk buttermilk (fat-free) *1 cup*	85

Food and Measures	Approximate Calories
condensed....1½ tbs.	100
evaporated....½ cup (1 cup diluted)	160
instant non-fat dry 6 tbs.	80
skim milk, fresh 1 cup	85
whole milk....1 cup	170
yogurt, plain 1 cup	120–160
Mints, cream.... ½-in. cube	5
Molasses....1 tbs.	70
Muffins bran....1 medium	90
1-egg....1 medium	130
Mushrooms....10 large	10
Mustard greens ½ cup, cooked	30

N

Noodles....¾ cup, cooked	75

O

Oatmeal.... ¾ cup, cooked	110
Oil—corn, cottonseed, olive, peanut, safflower 1 tbs.	100
Okra....10–15 pods	50
Olives Green....4 medium, or 3 extra large	15
Ripe....3 small, or 2 large	15
Onions....3–4 medium	100
Orange....1 medium	80
juice....1 cup	125
Oysters....5 medium	100

Food and Measures	Approximate Calories
P	
Parsnips....1 parsnip 7 ins. long	100
Peaches canned in syrup 2 lg. halves and 3 tbs. juice	100
dried....4 medium halves	100
fresh....1 medium	50
Peanut butter....1 tbs.	100
Peanuts, shelled....10	50
Pears canned in syrup 3 halves and 3 tbs. juice	100
fresh....1 medium	50
Peas canned....½ cup	65
fresh, shelled....¾ cup	100
Pecans....6	100
Pepper, green.... 1 medium	20
Pickles, cucumber sour and dill....10 slices 2 ins. in diam.	10
sweet....1 small	10
Pies....(sectors from 9-in pies) apple 3-in. sector	200
lemon meringue 3-in. sector	300
mincemeat 3-in. sector	300
pumpkin.... 3-in. sector	250
Pineapple canned, unsweetened 1 slice ½-in. thick and	

Food and Measures	Approximate Calories
1 tbs. juice	50
fresh....1 slice ¾-in. thick	50
juice, unsweetened 1 cup	135
Plums	
canned....2 med. and 1 tbs. juice	75
fresh....2 medium	50
Popcorn, plain....1½ cups, popped	100
Popovers....1 popover	100
Pork chop, lean 1 medium	200
Potato chips.... 8–10 large	100
Potato salad with mayonnaise.... ½ cup	200
Potatoes	
mashed....½ cup	100
sweet....½ medium	100
white....1 medium	100
Prune juice....½ cup	100
Prunes, dried.... 4 medium	100
Pumpkin....½ cup	50

R

Food and Measures	Approximate Calories
Radishes....5	10
Raisins....¼ cup	90
Raspberries, fresh.... 1 cup	90
Rhubarb, stewed and sweetened....½ cup	100
Rice....¾ cup, cooked	100
Roll, Parker House 1 medium	100
Rutabagas....½ cup	30

S

Food and Measures	Approximate Calories
Salad dressing	
boiled....1 tbs.	25
French....1 tbs.	90
mayonnaise....1 tbs.	100
Salmon, canned.... ½ cup	100
Sardines, drained....5 fish 3 ins. long	100
Sauerkraut....½ cup	15
Sherbet....½ cup	120
Soup, condensed....11-oz. can	
mushroom	360
noodle	290
tomato	230
vegetable	200
Spaghetti....¾ cup, cooked	100
Spinach....½ cup, cooked	20
Squash	
summer....½ cup, cooked	20
winter....½ cup, cooked	50
Strawberries, fresh.... 1 cup	90
Sugar	
brown....1 tbs.	50
granulated....1 tbs.	50
powdered....1 tbs.	40
Sweetbreads, calves; 1 pair med.-sized	200
Swiss chard ½ cup leaves and stems	30

T

Food and Measures	Approximate Calories
Tangerines....1 medium	60

Food and Measures	Approximate Calories
Tapioca, uncooked....1 tbs.	50
Tomato juice....1 cup	60
Tomatoes, canned.... ½ cup	25
fresh....1 medium	30
Tuna fish, canned ¼ cup, drained	100
Turkey, lean....1 slice 4 by 2½ by ¼ ins.	100
Turnip....1 turnip 1¾ ins. in diam.	25
Turnip greens....½ cup, cooked	30

V

Food and Measures	Approximate Calories
Veal, roast....1 slice 3 by 3¾ by ½ ins.	120

W

Food and Measures	Approximate Calories
Waffles....1 waffle 6 ins. in diam.	250

Food and Measures	Approximate Calories
Walnuts....8	100
Watermelon....1 round slice 6 ins. in diam. 1½ ins. thick, no rind	190
Wheat flakes....¾ cup	100
germ....1 tbs.	25
shredded....1 biscuit	100

* * *

Food and Measures	Approximate Calories
Alcoholic beverages beer....8 ozs.	120
gin....1½ ozs.	120
rum....1½ ozs.	150
whiskey....1½ ozs.	150
Wines champagne....4 ozs.	120
port....1 oz.	50
sherry....1 oz.	40
table, red or white 4 ozs.	95

Source: Metropolitan Life Insurance Company

SEVEN AIDS TO LOSING WEIGHT PERMANENTLY

1. *Cut down on extra hard fats.* Most people don't realize the high calorie count in that little bit of butter, those few fried potatoes, that handful of snacks. Cut down on foods that have hard or saturated fats.

2. *Eat meals in courses.* A cup of clear soup followed by a light entree, then a final course of a light dessert, is much more appetite-appeasing than the same number of calories served in one or two dishes.

3. *Think light, not heavy.* Rediscover the superb flavor of fresh fish, simply prepared with just a touch of lemon. Relish the seasonal delight of fresh aspara-

gus, the delicious taste of broiled chicken, the elegance of fresh fruit for dessert. You can eat with pleasure while eating light.

4. *Get to know the approximate calories in those high-calorie foods you like best, as well as those that are calorie-low.* This way, if nothing will satisfy you but well-buttered corn on the cob, you can have it. You can then compensate with a second very low-calorie vegetable and a lower-calorie meat or fish. For example, would anyone ever complain about the calorie cost of a cook-out? Not with this menu: corn on cob, fresh tomatoes, broiled fish and fresh fruit. See what we mean? (See calorie chart in this chapter.)

5. *Watch those between-meal snacks.* Just a few high-calorie cookies can wreck your calorie count. Try low-calorie snacks before you decide "it won't matter just this once."

6. *Do eat desserts.* You won't be nearly so tempted to indulge in second helpings if a sweet is to follow. Honey is a good appetite-pleaser on cut-up fresh fruit. A delicious, healthful, natural dessert, small though it may be, leaves you feeling pleasantly full without overeating.

7. *Finally, don't get discouraged if you fail to lose as quickly as you would like.* Consistent weight loss, no matter how little each week, will eventually do the job. And what is really important is that it will probably stay lost.

EXERCISE CAN MELT CALORIES

Weight depends not only on how many calories are taken in during the day, but also on how many are used up in physical activity. The fat person who

131

merely cuts down his intake of food to lose weight will make slow progress since the number of calories needed to maintain the body is much smaller than most people think.

If you add just 30 minutes of moderate exercise to your daily schedule, you can lose about 25 pounds in one year. An exercise should be sufficiently vigorous to use up the required number of calories, and to some degree, it must be sustained. Remember, that although it takes one hour of jogging to use up 900 calories, you do not have to do it all at once; a half-hour, for example, uses up 450 calories. It is a fact that you must walk 35 miles to lose one pound of fat . . . but the 35 miles need not be walked at one time.

Walking one additional mile each day for 35 days also will take off that pound. So keep walking, keep active, and use up the excess calories.

It is true that steady, moderate exercise or activ-

EXERCISE-ACTIVITY TABLE

	Calories Per Hour		Calories Per Hour
Bicycling	300–420	Ping Pong	360
Bowling	260	Running	800–1,000
Dancing	450–700	Skating	300–700
Gardening	350	Skiing	600
Golf	210–300	Swimming	350–700
Housework	180–240	Tennis	400–500
Horseback Riding	180–480	Volleyball	210
Ice Skating	360	Walking	100–330

This chart is based on studies reported by the American Heart Association and the Nutrition Foundation.

ities will burn up small amounts of extra calories. Over a period of time, these small losses add up to a loss of extra unwanted pounds. What is more, such exercise will stimulate your circulation, dissipate tension and loosen joints. It will also add muscle tone and give a general feeling of well-being. More tips to help bring down overweight:

Weigh yourself once a week and keep a written record of your progress. Don't be surprised if there are times when the scales fail to show a loss even when you have been faithful to your diet. Lost fat is sometimes replaced *temporarily* with water in the tissues. This condition gradually corrects itself as dieting continues.

Be sure to eat a good breakfast; it should supply from one-fourth to one-third of your total daily calories. This not only gives you needed nourishment, but makes it easier to resist the temptation to snack between meals, or eat too much lunch.

Eat meals slowly, allowing time for the blood sugar to rise. This helps make smaller amounts of food more satisfying.

If you are hungry before mealtime, a cup of clear bouillon, tomato juice or even a glass of water can help. Or munch on celery, carrots or radishes.

If you are in the habit of having a snack while reading or watching television, save the dessert or beverage from lunch or dinner for snack-time. Or try raw vegetables, a small fresh fruit, grapefruit or tomato juice.

Dry skimmed milk can substitute for whole milk in any cooked dish.

Lemon juice, not butter, is a slim gourmet's choice for seasoning steamed vegetables.

Potatoes, mashed with skim-milk cottage cheese

plus a bit of parmesan cheese, have it, flavor-wise, all over mashed-with-butter-and-cream.

A vegetable soufflé—carrots, mushroom or spinach, for instance—is deceptively filling. Used as a satisfying main course, it is a great calorie saver.

A doctor-approved weight means you will also bring down extra high blood pressure. Finally, remember that if you want to keep your weight down, you should keep your stomach comfortable at all times. Eat three balanced meals a day. You cannot skip breakfast. You cannot skip lunch. You may set aside a few calories from each meal for a safe snack in between. This will keep your satiety level high, and prevent you from craving food.

CHAPTER ELEVEN

QUESTIONS AND ANSWERS ABOUT HIGH BLOOD PRESSURE

HERE IS A GENERAL SUMMATION OF THE HEALTH problem of high blood pressure, in question and answer form:

What is blood pressure?

It is the force of the blood against the walls of arteries. The pressure is greatest at the moment blood is pumped by the left ventricle.

How is blood pressure measured?

A sphygmomanometer (pronounced sfig-mo-mah-nom-e-ter) is used. It has several parts. One part is a bandage-like cloth—a cuff—that will hold air. It is wrapped around your arm. A rubber tube connects the cuff to a pressure meter. The doctor uses a squeeze bulb to pump air into the cuff. He slowly releases the air and uses a stethoscope to listen to the blood in your arm. When he first hears the sound of the heart pumping, he reads the meter. He reads the meter again when the sound disappears.

What is normal blood pressure?

The normal reading when the heart pumps is 100 to 140. This is *systolic pressure.* When the heart rests, the normal reading is between 70 and 90. This is *diastolic pressure.*

How is blood pressure written?

The systolic pressure is written first, then the diastolic pressure. Examples are: 140/80 or 130/74. These are read: "140 over 80" or "130 over 74." Both of these pressures fall within normal range.

Does blood pressure change?

Yes. It goes up when you are excited, afraid or tense. It goes down when you are relaxed or sleeping. These changes are considered normal.

What happens if your blood pressure is high all the time?

Doctors call this *hypertension,* or high blood pressure. It may be serious because it makes the heart work harder.

What, specifically, is high blood pressure?

It's blood pressure that is too high all the time. Blood pressure normally goes up and down. If you have a high blood pressure reading once or twice, don't worry. It doesn't necessarily mean hypertension. But have it checked regularly.

What causes hypertension?

No one knows what causes the most common type. For a long time, no one thought that tension really had anything to do with it. But now, it is believed that tension may be a factor in the most common type of hypertension. A family tendency may also be a factor.

What are the typical symptoms of high blood pressure?

This is the big problem of the ailment—its lack of symptoms. Typically, in the early stages a hypertensive feels fine. Although headache, easy fatigue, shortness of breath and dizziness can occur with high blood pressure, they also occur in many other disorders. Be sure to obtain regular examinations.

Is high blood pressure serious?

Yes, it often is. It makes the artery walls hard and thick. It also takes away the elastic stretchiness that is important to arteries. This affects the heart. Once the stretch is gone, the heart must work harder to pump enough blood. If this goes on for a long time, the heart itself may get larger. This condition is called *hypertensive heart disease.* High blood pressure also can cause a stroke. The extra force of the blood may break an artery in the brain. If that happens, a *cerebral hemorrhage* occurs.

Can heredity be a factor contributing to hypertension?

A tendency toward hypertension runs in families, but the condition often skips family members, or a whole generation or more. Therefore, it is not invariably inherited but this factor can not be ruled out.

What are the factors involving age and sex?

In general, blood pressure rises with age. The onset of hypertension, however, is usually found in early middle age. More men than women under age 50 are susceptible to hypertension. In older age groups, more women than men have high blood pressure.

Is overweight a factor?

Generally speaking, people who are overweight tend to have higher blood pressure than those of normal weight.

Can tension and anxiety raise blood pressure?

Yes, living situations that create stress do bring

on higher blood pressure. However, a certain amount of stress is not necessarily harmful, provided it is resolved quickly; for example the stress caused by the problems of daily living. Prolonged and unresolved stress is more likely to bring on hypertension.

Is smoking harmful?

Heavy cigarette smoking is often implicated in hypertension. Nicotine is known to constrict blood vessels and therefore increase blood pressure and pulse rate.

What if hypertension goes untreated?

The condition usually persists and may get worse. Hypertension causes the heart to pump with extra force and subjects the blood vessels to ever-increasing pressure. The heart tends to enlarge when it must work harder than normal over a long period. In time, these stresses and strains may seriously affect the entire circulatory system.

What can hypertension do to the arteries?

The arteries and arterioles (small arteries) or blood vessels, tend to harden after years of hypertension. They become narrower and less flexible. Most people develop some hardening of the arteries anyway as they grow older, but hypertension pushes the process along a little faster.

Does hypertension always lead directly to a stroke?

It is not a hard and fast rule. Of course, a stroke can occur in someone with hypertension, but only a small percentage of hypertensive persons have strokes.

What can be done to ease the problems?

Try to minimize tension, anxiety and stress. While it may be impossible to be free from worry, it is possible to avoid undue emotional strain and tension. It may be easier said than done, but you should try to shield yourself from stress situations. It will help your condition.

Is exercise beneficial?

Exercise releases tension. But avoid strenuous activities that you are not used to. Your physician should decide the pace and type of activities best for you.

Is sleep helpful?

Very much so! Blood pressure goes down during sleep. Therefore, a good night's sleep and a short nap in the afternoon are important.

Is there a high blood pressure "type" of individual?

Generally speaking, no. It is a popular misconception that the hypertensive is nervous, compulsive, a never-resting perfectionist who cannot sit still. This is not a typical picture, although it may fit some hypertensives. Some people with high blood pressure are relaxed, well-adjusted and quiet.

What effect does high blood pressure have on the kidneys?

The kidneys begin to suffer as pressure damages the tiny arteries in these organs. Eventually the kidneys fail to filter the waste products and sickness and death can follow.

What may eventually happen if treatment for high blood pressure is not followed?

There are three risks: (1) The kidneys may fail. (2) Brain hemorrhage can occur. (3) The heart, unable to stand prolonged strain, may fail.

If I am placed on a low sodium diet, will there be a potassium deficiency?

Often a doctor will prescribe a low sodium diet and a diuretic drug. This removes salt from the body.

Naturally, the drug removes other substances, such as potassium. People who take digitalis, a heart drug, may run the risk of abnormal heart rhythms. The doctor will frequently recommend potassium supplements. Ordinarily a food program contains from 1050 to 2050 milligrams of sodium daily as compared to 1400 to 6050 milligrams of potassium daily. Potassium food supplements are easily available, but leave it up to your doctor. You should also consider eating foods with potassium content in the amounts approved by your physician. The chart on page 141 lists the potassium content of everyday foods.

In one year, high blood pressure can end the lives of about 250,000 Americans. That is one out of eight of every one who will die from anything. Some 23 million people have high blood pressure. That is one in every ten adults. Don't take chances. Get your blood pressure taken. Follow the procedure your physician advises so that you can enjoy normal blood pressure and a healthy, long life.

POTASSIUM CONTENT OF SELECTED FOODS

Food	Quantity	Potassium Content (mg app.)
Meats		
Hamburger	3 oz.	290
Beef Chuck	3 oz.	310
Beef Round	3 oz.	340
Rib Roast	3 oz.	290
Chicken Fryer	4 oz.	710
Turkey	4 oz.	350
Vegetables		
Sweet Corn	1 cup	230
Lima Beans	1 cup	520
Tomato	1 med.	340
Brussels Sprouts	1 cup	300
Spinach	1 cup	600
Artichoke	1 med.	210
Fruits		
Banana	1 med.	630
Orange	1 med.	360
Apricots	3 med.	500
Dates	1 cup	1390
Cantaloupe	½ melon	880
Raisins	1 cup	1150
Grapefruit	1 cup	380
Watermelon	½ slice	380
Peach	1 med.	180
Juice		
Orange	8 oz.	440
Grapefruit	8 oz.	370
Prune	8 oz.	620
Pineapple	8 oz.	340

Source: American Pharmaceutical Association
James Mckenney. "Antihypertensive Drug Therapy." *Journal of the American Pharmaceutical Association*: April, 1974, 208, 209.

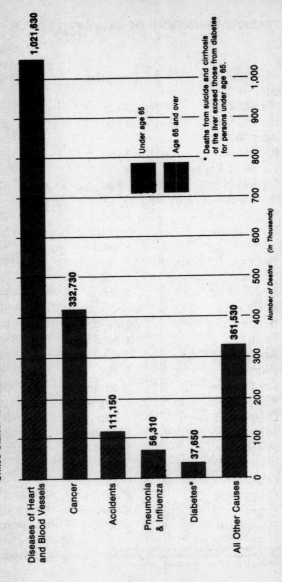

Leading Causes of Death
United States: 1971 Estimates

Diseases of Heart and Blood Vessels — 1,021,630
Cancer — 332,730
Accidents — 111,150
Pneumonia & Influenza — 56,310
Diabetes* — 37,650
All Other Causes — 361,530

Under age 65
Age 65 and over

* Deaths from suicide and cirrhosis of the liver exceed those from diabetes for persons under age 65.

Number of Deaths (In Thousands)

0 100 200 300 400 500 600 700 800 900 1,000

Source: National Center for Health Statistics, U.S. Public Health Service, DHEW and The American Heart Association

GLOSSARY OF WORDS YOUR DOCTOR MAY USE

A

ADIPOSE TISSUE—Fatty tissue, widely distributed throughout the body

ADRENAL GLANDS—A pair of endocrine glands that sit atop the kidneys. The inner portion of each gland, the adrenal medulla, secretes norepinephrine and epinephrine, both powerful heart stimulants and blood-vessel constrictors. The outer shell, or adrenal cortex, secretes aldosterone, cortisone and other steroidal hormones that influence the metabolism of salt, water, carbohydrates, etc.

ALDOSTERONE—A hormone secreted by the adrenal cortex that promotes the conservation of salt and water by the kidneys

ANGINA PECTORIS—Pain in the chest, and often in the left arm and shoulder, resulting from an insufficient blood supply to the heart muscle. Angina pectoris is usually caused by the narrowing of the coronary arteries by atherosclerosis. Attacks of chest pain are often brought on by exertion, fright or other stresses

ANGIOCARDIOGRAPHY—X-ray examination of the heart

and great blood vessels by tracing the course of a radiopaque fluid which has been injected into the blood stream

ANGIOTENSIN—A powerful blood-vessel constrictor generated from a protein in the blood through the action of renin, an enzyme released from the kidneys. Generated in excessive amounts when blood deprivation, disease or other factors cause the kidney to release increased quantities of renin, angiotensin is the initiator of renal hypertension

ANTICOAGULANTS—Drugs that delay clotting of the blood. When a blood vessel is plugged up by a clot, the drugs tend to prevent new clots from forming, or the existing clots from enlarging; they do not dissolve an existing clot. Examples are heparin and the coumarin derivatives

ANTIHYPERTENSIVE AGENTS—Drugs that are used to lower blood pressure, such as tranquilizers, drugs that relax blood vessels and diuretics, among others

AORTA—The main trunk artery which receives blood from the lower left chamber of the heart

ARRHYTHMIA—An abnormal rhythm of the heartbeat

ARTERIOLES—The smallest arterial vessels (about 0.2 mm. or 1/125 inch in diameter), the end branches of the arteries. They conduct the blood from the arteries to the capillaries. Generalized constriction of these vessels is a major factor in hypertension

ARTERIOSCLEROSIS—Commonly called hardening of the arteries. This is a generic term which includes the variety of conditions that cause artery walls to become thick and hard and lose elasticity

ARTERIES—Blood vessels that carry blood away from the heart to the various parts of the body. They carry oxygenated blood except for the pulmonary artery which carries unoxygenated blood from the heart to the lungs for oxygenation

ATRIUM—One of the two upper chambers of the heart. Also called auricle

ATHEROSCLEROSIS—A form of arteriosclerosis in which fatty deposits make the inner layer of the artery walls thick and irregular. These deposits (called atheromata) project above the surface of the inner layer of the artery, and thus decrease the diameter of the internal channel of the vessel

AUTONOMIC NERVOUS SYSTEM—Sometimes called the involuntary or vegetative nervous system, it regulates tissues and functions not under conscious control (heart beat, blood pressure, etc.). It consists of the sympathetic and parasympathetic nervous systems. These have opposing effects on the cardiovascular system: sympathetic stimuli tend to increase heart rate, constrict blood vessels and raise blood pressure; parasympathetic stimuli reduce heart rate, relax blood vessels and lower blood pressure

B

BARORECEPTORS—Aggregations of specialized, pressure-sensitive nerve cells. In the cardiovascular system, baroreceptors detect unusual rises and falls in blood pressure and act through the autonomic nervous system to stabilize blood pressure within normal limits

BLOOD PRESSURE—The pressure of the blood in the arteries.
1. Systolic blood pressure. Blood pressure when the heart muscle is contracted (systole)
2. Diastolic blood pressure. Blood pressure when the heart muscle is relaxed between beats (diastole). Blood pressure is generally expressed by two numbers, as 120/80, the first representing the systolic, and the second, the diastolic pressure

BLOOD VOLUME—The amount of blood circulating

within the body. In normal adults of average weight blood volume is about eight pints

"BLUE BABIES"—Babies who have a blueness of skin (cyanosis) resulting from insufficient oxygen in the arterial blood, often indicating a heart defect

BRACHIAL ARTERY—The chief artery of the upper arm

C

CADMIUM—A non-essential trace metal, present in minute quantities in many foods and beverages, that tends to accumulate in the kidneys. Preliminary evidence suggests that this accumulation may be a factor in the development of hypertension

CAPILLARIES—Extremely narrow tubes forming a network between the arterioles and the veins. The walls are composed of a single layer of cells through which oxygen and nutritive materials pass out to the tissues. Carbon dioxide and waste products are admitted from the tissues into the blood stream

CARDIAC—Pertaining to the heart

CARDIAC ARREST—When the heart stops beating; the cessation of cardiac output and effective circulation

CARDIOPULMONARY RESUSCITATION—A combination of chest compression and mouth-to-mouth breathing. Used during fibrillation or cardiac arrest to keep oxygenated blood flowing to the brain until appropriate medical treatment can be initiated

CARDIOVASCULAR—Pertaining to the heart and blood vessels

CAROTID ARTERIES—The left and right common carotid arteries are the principal arteries supplying blood to the head and neck. Each has two main branches, the external carotid artery and the internal carotid artery

CAROTID SINUS—A slight dilation at the point where

the internal carotid artery branches from the common carotid artery. The carotid arteries supply blood to the head and neck. The carotid sinus contains special nerve end organs which respond to a change in blood pressure by causing a change in the rate of heart beat. External pressure on the carotid sinus, by stimulating some of the nerves in the sinus, can also cause a drop in blood pressure and faintness

CATHETERIZATION—The process of examining the heart by introducing a thin tube (catheter) into a vein or artery and passing it into the heart

CENTRAL NERVOUS SYSTEM—In vertebrates, the brain and spinal cord. It receives sensory stimuli, transmits motor stimuli, and supervises and coordinates the activity of the entire nervous system

CEREBRAL THROMBOSIS—Formation of a blood clot in a blood vessel leading to the brain

CEREBROVASCULAR ACCIDENT—Also called cerebral vascular accident, apoplexy or stroke. An impeded blood supply to some part of the brain

CEREBROVASCULAR DISEASE—Pertaining to diseases of the blood vessels in the brain

CHOLESTEROL—A fat-like substance found in animal tissue. In blood tests the normal level for young, healthy Americans is between 180 and 230 milligrams per 100 cc. Higher levels are associated with increasing age and risk of coronary atherosclerosis

CINEANGIOGRAPHY—The taking of moving pictures to show the passage of an opaque dye through blood vessels

CIRCULATORY SYSTEM—Pertaining to the heart, blood vessels and the circulation of the blood

COARCTATION OF THE AORTA—One of the several types of congenital heart defects. Literally a pressing together or narrowing of the aorta

COLLATERAL CIRCULATION—The heart's own life-saving method. A system of smaller blood vessels carry blood when a main blood vessel is blocked

CONGENITAL DEFECTS—Malformations of the heart or its major blood vessels present at birth

CONGESTIVE HEART FAILURE—A backing up of blood in the veins leading to the heart often accompanied by accumulation of fluid in various parts of the body. It results from the heart's inability to pump out all the blood that returns to it

CONSTRICTION—Narrowing of the internal diameter of blood vessels, caused by a contraction of the muscular coat of the vessels

CORONARY ARTERIES—Two arteries, arising from the aorta, arching down over the top of the heart and conducting blood to the heart muscle

CORONARY ATHEROSCLEROSIS—An irregular thickening of the inner layer of the walls of the arteries that conduct blood to the heart muscle. The internal channel of these arteries (the coronaries) becomes narrowed, and the blood supply to the heart muscle is reduced

CORONARY CARE UNIT—An in-hospital or emergency mobile unit, equipped with monitoring devices and staffed with trained personnel, designed to treat coronary patients

CORONARY HEART DISEASE—Atherosclerosis of the coronary arteries that supply blood to the heart muscle itself; it is the blood-vessel disease usually underlying angina pectoris and most heart attacks

CORONARY OCCLUSION—An obstruction or narrowing of one of the coronary arteries which hinders the blood flow to some part of the heart muscle. (See Heart Attack)

CORONARY THROMBOSIS—Formation of a clot in one of the arteries which conduct blood to the heart muscle. Also called coronary occlusion

CYANOSIS—Blueness of skin caused by insufficient oxygen in the blood

D

DEFIBRILLATOR—An agent or measure which stops an incoordinate contraction of the heart muscle and reestablishes normal rhythm

DIABETES—A chronic disorder of carbohydrate metabolism due to a disturbance of the normal insulin mechanism

DIASTOLIC PRESSURE—The blood pressure level during the time the heart muscle is relaxed

DIGITALIS—A drug which strengthens the contraction of the heart muscle, slows the rate of contraction of the heart and promotes the elimination of fluid from body tissues

DILATION—Enlargement of blood vessels, usually through the relaxation of muscle fibers in the blood-vessel wall

DIURETIC—A drug that promotes the excretion of urine

E

EDEMA—Swelling caused by abnormally large amounts of fluid in the body tissues

ELECTROCARDIOGRAM—A graphic record of the electric current produced by the heart

ELECTROLYTE—Any substance that, in solution, is capable of conducting electricity by means of its atoms or groups of atoms, and in the process breaks down into positively and negatively charged particles. Examples: sodium or potassium

EMBOLUS—A blood clot that forms in the blood vessels in one part of the body and travels to another

ENDOCRINE GLANDS—The glands that secrete hormones distributed in the body by way of the bloodstream.

They include the pituitary, thyroid, parathyroids, adrenals, testes, ovaries, thymus and pancreas

ENVIRONMENT—Surroundings. The aggregate of all external conditions and influences affecting the life and development of an organism

ENZYME—A complex organic substance capable of speeding up specific biochemical processes in the body. Enzymes are universally present in living organisms

EPINEPHRINE—One of the secretions of two small glands, the adrenal glands, located just above the kidneys. This powerful stimulant, also called adrenaline, constricts the small blood vessels (arterioles), increases the rate of heart beat and raises blood pressure

ESSENTIAL HYPERTENSION—Sometimes called primary hypertension, and commonly known as high blood pressure. An elevated blood pressure not caused by kidney or other evident disease

F

FIBRILLATION—Uncoordinated contractions of the heart muscle occurring when individual muscle fibers take up independent irregular contractions

FIBRIN—The substance which enmeshes blood corpuscles in the blood-clotting mechanism

G

GANGLION—A mass of nerve cells, which serves as a center of nervous influence

GANGLIONIC BLOCKING AGENTS—A drug that blocks the transmission of a nerve impulse at the nerve centers (ganglia). Some of these drugs, such as hexamethonium and mecamylamine hydrochloride, may be used in the treatment of high blood pressure

GUANETHIDINE—An extremely potent agent used for the treatment of moderate to severe hypertension

H

HEART ATTACK—A coronary occlusion or obstruction (generally a blood clot) in one of the coronary arteries that reduces or stops the flow of blood to some area of the heart muscle (myocardium) and results in damage to or death of that area. (See Myocardial Infarction)

HEART-LUNG MACHINE—An apparatus through which the blood stream is diverted for pumping and oxygenating while the stilled heart is opened for surgery

HEREDITY—Genetic transmission of the physical and constitutional traits of parents to their offspring

HIGH BLOOD PRESSURE (HYPERTENSION)—An unstable or persistent elevation of blood pressure above the normal range

HOMOGRAFT—A graft of tissue taken from the body of another person

HORMONE—A secretion of an endocrine gland that has a specific effect on the activities of other organs

HYPERTENSION—Commonly called high blood pressure. An unstable or persistent elevation of blood pressure above the normal range, that may eventually lead to increased heart size and kidney damage

HYPOTENSION—Commonly called low blood pressure. Blood pressure below the normal range. Most commonly used to describe an acute fall in blood pressure, as occurs in shock

HYPOXIA—Less than normal content of oxygen in the organs and tissues of the body

I

INCIDENCE—The number of new cases of a disease

developing in a given population during a specified period of time

K
KIDNEY—One of a pair of bean-shaped organs situated in the body cavity near the spinal column. Excretory functions include removal via the urine of urea, uric acid and other waste products of metabolism. The kidneys are also vital to the maintenance of the internal environment of the body through the regulation of fluid, electrolyte and acid-base balance

M
METHYL DOPA—Drug used to combat moderate to severe hypertension

MONOAMINE OXIDASE—One of two enzymes chiefly responsible for inactivating norepinephrine in the body (the other is called catechol-o-methyl transferase)

MORTALITY RATE—The number of deaths from a specific cause that occurred in a unit of population (such as per 100,000 or per 10,000 or per 1,000) in a specified time, such as a year

MYOCARDIAL INFARCTION—The damaging or death of an area of the heart muscle (myocardium) resulting from a reduction in the blood supply reaching that area

MYOCARDIUM—The muscular wall of the heart which contracts in order to pump blood out of the heart and then relaxes as the heart refills with returning blood

N
NEUROHORMONE—A chemical substance manufactured and stored in nerve tissue. It is released by

nerve impulses to bridge the slight gaps called synapses that exist between nerves at nerve junctions and between nerve endings and their target organs. Two major neurohormones are acetylcholine and norepinephrine

NITROGLYCERIN—Drug which causes dilation of blood vessels, often used in the treatment of angina pectoris

NOREPINEPHRINE—An organic compound, also called noradrenalin and levarterenol, which is a potent heart stimulant and blood-vessel constrictor. A neurohormone acting between sympathetic nerve endings and target organs, norepinephrine is also released into the blood from the adrenal glands during exertion, fright or stress. It is often used medically in the treatment of shock

O

OBESITY—A condition marked by excessive deposition and storage of fat in the body; corpulence; overweight

OCCLUDED ARTERY—One in which blood flow has been impaired by a blockage

OPEN HEART SURGERY—Surgery performed on the opened heart while the blood stream is diverted through a heart-lung machine

P

PARAMEDICAL—Pertaining or closely related to the art and practice of medicine. Personnel whose work supports, or is closely related to that of practicing physicians

PARASYMPATHETIC NERVOUS SYSTEM—One of two opposing divisions of the autonomic or involuntary nervous system. In the cardiovascular system, the effects of parasympathetic stimulation slow the heart rate and reduce its output of blood, relax blood vessels and reduce blood pressure

PARGYLINE—A drug used in moderate to severe cases of hypertension

PATENT DUCTUS ARTERIOSUS—A congenital defect; the fetal ductus arteriosus (an opening between the aorta and the pulmonary artery) does not close after birth

PHEOCHROMOCYTOMA—A tumor which arises in the adrenal glands. It produces and releases into the blood large quantities of norepinephrine and epinephrine. These powerful stimulants produce such symptoms of pheochromocytoma as hypertension, elevated heart rate, headaches, anxiety, and excessive sweating

POLYUNSATURATED FAT—A fat so constituted chemically that it is capable of absorbing additional hydrogen. These fats are usually liquid oils of vegetable origin, such as corn oil or safflower oil. A diet with a high polyunsaturated fat content tends to lower the amount of cholesterol in the blood. These fats are recommended as partial substitutes for saturated fat in a diet to lessen the rate of accumulation of fatty deposits in the arteries

POTASSIUM—A mineral whose compounds are present in many foods and beverages, potassium is absolutely essential to life and health. It is the major electrolyte of the fluid inside body cells and is essential in many functions, such as the transmission of nerve impulses, the contraction of muscle, and others

PREVALENCE—The number of cases of a given disease in a given population at a specified moment of time

PRIMARY HYPERTENSION—Sometimes called essential hypertension, and commonly known as high blood pressure. An elevated blood pressure not caused by kidney or other evident disease

PROPHYLAXIS—Preventive treatment
PROSTHETICS—Artificial substitutes for missing parts
PULMONARY—Pertaining to the lungs

R
RENAL—Pertaining to the kidneys
RENAL HYPERTENSION—High blood pressure caused by damage to or diseases of the kidneys. The most common cause of renal hypertension is atherosclerotic deposits or other obstructions to normal kidney bloodflow. The blood-deprived kidney releases renin, an enzyme that acts on a plasma protein to give rise to angiotensin, a powerful blood vessel constrictor that initiates renal hypertension
RESERPINE—One of the organic substances found in the root of the plant, *rauwolfia serpentina,* which lowers blood pressure, slows the heart rate, and has tranquilizing and sedative effects. One of the antihypertensive agents
RETINA—The sensory membrane that lines most of the posterior chamber of the eye, receives the image formed by the lens, is the immediate instrument of vision and is connected to the brain by the optic nerve
RHEUMATIC FEVER—A disease, usually occurring in childhood, which may follow a streptococcal infection
RHEUMATIC HEART DISEASE—The damage done to the heart, particularly the heart valves, by one or more attacks of rheumatic fever
RUBELLA—Commonly known as German measles

S
SATURATED FAT—A fat so constituted chemically that it is not capable of absorbing any more hydrogen.

These are usually the solid fats of animal origin such as the fats in milk, butter, meat, etc. A diet high in saturated fat content tends to increase the amount of cholesterol in the blood. These fats are restricted in the diet to lessen the deposition of fatty particles in the blood vessels

SCLEROSIS—This applies to a process that develops in arteries or arterioles. It is a scarring and thickening of the walls. In arteries it is called "hardening"; in arterioles, whose openings are so small in relation to the thickness of the walls, it tends to close off the openings completely. Hypertension causes arteriosclerosis or accelerates other types of sclerosis

SECONDARY HYPERTENSION—An elevated blood pressure caused by (i.e., secondary to) certain specific diseases or infections

SEDATIVE—A drug that depresses the activity of the central nervous system, thus having a calming effect. Examples are barbiturates, chloral hydrate and bromides

SEPTUM—The muscular walls dividing the two chambers on the left side of the heart from the two on the right

SODIUM—A mineral essential to life, found in nearly all plant and animal tissue. Table salt (sodium chloride) is nearly half sodium. It is the major electrolyte of blood and other extracellular fluids. In some types of heart disease the body retains an excess of sodium and water, and therefore sodium intake is restricted

SPHYGMOMANOMETER—An instrument that measures blood pressure in the arteries

STETHOSCOPE—An instrument for listening to sounds within the body

"STREP" INFECTION (STREPTOCOCCAL INFECTION)—An

infection, usually in the throat resulting from the presence of streptococcus

STROKE (ALSO CALLED APOPLEXY, CEREBROVASCULAR ACCIDENT OR CEREBRAL VASCULAR ACCIDENT)—An impeded blood supply to some part of the brain

SYMPATHETIC NERVOUS SYSTEM—One of two opposing divisions of the autonomic nervous system, which regulates functions not under voluntary control. In the cardiovascular system, sympathetic stimulation increases heart rate and its output of blood, constricts blood vessels and raises blood pressure

SYMPATHECTOMY—An operation that interrupts some part of the sympathetic nervous system. The sympathetic nervous system is a part of the autonomic or involuntary nervous system and normally regulates tissues not under voluntary control, e.g., glands, heart and smooth muscles. Sometimes the interruption is accomplished by drugs, in which case it is called a chemical sympathectomy

SYSTEMIC CIRCULATION—The circulation of the blood through all parts of the body except the lungs, the flow being from the left lower chamber of the heart (left ventricle) through the body and back to the right upper chamber of the heart (right atrium)

SYSTOLIC BLOOD PRESSURE—Pressure inside the arteries when the heart contracts at each beat

T

TERMINAL STORES—The quantities of a neurohormone (e.g., norepinephrine) kept on tap in the nerve endings for release, as needed, by nerve impulses to convey their directives to target organs

THERAPEUTIC AGENT—A drug used to treat a disease or to control its symptoms

THIAZIDE DIURETICS—A family of drugs that increases the excretion of sodium by the kidneys and thereby promotes increased water elimination. These drugs are often used to combat excessive fluid retention and edema. They also produce modest blood pressure reductions and support the effectiveness of other blood-pressure-reducing drugs, and so are often used in the treatment of hypertension

THROMBOSIS—The formation or presence of a blood clot (thrombus) inside a blood vessel or cavity of the heart

THROMBUS—A blood clot which forms inside a blood vessel or cavity of the heart

TRANQUILIZER—A drug that exerts a calming effect by reducing the activity of the central nervous system. Some tranquilizers, notably reserpine, are also effective agents for reducing blood pressure in hypertension

V

VASCULAR—Pertaining to the blood vessels

VEIN—Any one of a series of vessels of the vascular system which carries blood from various parts of the body back to the heart. All veins in the body conduct unoxygenated blood except the pulmonary veins which conduct freshly oxygenated blood from the lungs back to the heart

VENTRICLE—One of the two lower chambers of the heart